Dr. Susan Lark's

The Menopause Self Help Book

A WOMAN'S GUIDE TO FEELING WONDERFUL FOR THE SECOND HALF OF HER LIFE

Susan M. Lark, M.D.

The first completely practical all-natural master plan to relieve and prevent every symptom of menopause

---

CELESTIALARTS

Berkeley, California

To my wonderful husband Jim, thank you for all your help. And to my darling daughter Rebecca, thanks for being so much fun.

CELESTIAL ARTS
P.O. Box 7327
Berkeley, California 94707

Cover design by Ken Scott
Photographs by Pete Macchia
Composition by Wilsted & Taylor
Illustrations © 1990 by Ellen Joy Sasaki

Library of Congress Cataloging-in-Publication Data
Lark, Susan M., 1945–
    The menopause self help book / Susan M. Lark.
        p.224 cm
    Includes bibliographical references.
    ISBN 0-89087-592-8
    1. Menopause—Popular works.   2. Middle aged women—Health and
hygiene.   I. Title.
RG186.L37   1990
618.1'75—dc20   89-25292 CIP

First Printing, 1990

     7   8   9   10   —   96   95   94

Manufactured in the United States of America

Contents

A Self Help Approach to Menopause

I have written this self help book on menopause for the more than fifty million American women over the age of fifty and the millions more between the ages of 35 and 49. Since I am currently in my late forties, I share the same concerns about remaining strong and healthy as I go through menopause and beyond. All of us want to minimize the symptoms and discomforts of menopause and to slow down the aging process. We want to continue to be productive and enjoy our later years with vigor and vitality.

For many women, however, an easy and symptom-free menopause is not what they experience at all. Many women in their thirties and forties have an increase in premenstrual tension, menstrual irregularities and a decrease in fertility as they move towards menopause. By the time they are fifty, most women have ceased menstruating entirely. The sharp decrease in their hormonal levels that occurs with menopause causes a new set of problems, including such health concerns as hot flashes, night sweats, mood swings, and thinning of the bones. The incidence of other health problems, such as heart disease and cancer, begins to accelerate.

Many of these menopause-related symptoms and health problems can be prevented, or at least minimized, through proper self help techniques. These techniques, which include specific dietary guidelines for menopausal women, as well as the right nutritional supplements, exercise programs, and stress-reduction techniques, can have dramatic beneficial effects for women in mid-life and beyond. Unfortunately, most of this exciting information lies buried in medical research journals and has not been made available for the women who need it.

While many books have been written about menopause, they have primarily discussed the symptoms of menopause and the standard hormonal treatments. There has been little in-depth information available on what mid-life women can do on their own to maintain their health and well-being. I have written this book to fill the need that women have for more complete self help information.

For almost two decades I have worked with thousands of women who were in their pre- and post-menopausal years. All of my patients have had an intense desire for information on how to stay healthy and symptom-free. All of this self help information is now available in this book, and I hope you will find it as useful as my patients have. I practice these techniques, too. Preventive health care has had tremendous benefits for me; I am healthier and more productive now than I was seven years ago. I plan to feel better and to be even healthier ten years from now. I am continually expanding my own knowledge about menopause self help and constantly researching new health care techniques.

How to Use the Menopause Self Help Book

A menopause self help program is important for all women. You will gain significant benefits from this program whether you are on hormonal therapy or not. To give you a wide range of options, I have included many self help techniques. A treatment plan that utilizes only one method and purports to be the only treatment for menopause will probably work for only a small percentage of women. In my own medical practice, I have found that results are much better if I completely individualize each patient's treatment program. By overlapping treatments from various disciplines, most women find a combination that works for them. There will be a combination that works for you, too.

This program is set up so that you can develop your own treatment plan. All the methods you need are contained in this book. They include nutrition, stress reduction, exercise, acupressure massage, pressure point exercises, and yoga. I have also included a great deal of information on vitamins, minerals, and herbs for menopause. Nutritional supplementation is a very important part of an optimal health program for women in the menopause years. Read through the entire book first to familiarize yourself with the material. The Menopause Workbook (Chapter 3) will help you evaluate your symptoms, and the Complete Treatment Chart for Menopause (Chapter 3) will tell you which treatments to use for your particular set of symptoms. Together they are quick and easy to use and will save you countless hours of work on your own. I have also included information on estrogen replacement therapy, which has long been the traditional medical treatment for menopause. To help you make your own decision about whether to use estrogen replacement therapy, I have included a chapter (Chapter 15) that includes a complete review of both the positive and negative aspects of estrogen use.

What will work for you can be found simply and quickly: try all of the therapies listed under your symptoms, and you will probably find that some make you feel better than others. Establish a regimen that works for you and use it every day. This program is practical and easy to follow. It can be used by itself or in conjunction with a medical program. And best of all, it works. The feeling of wellness that can be yours with a self help program will radiate out and touch your whole life. You will have more time and energy to enjoy your work, family, and other pleasures in life.

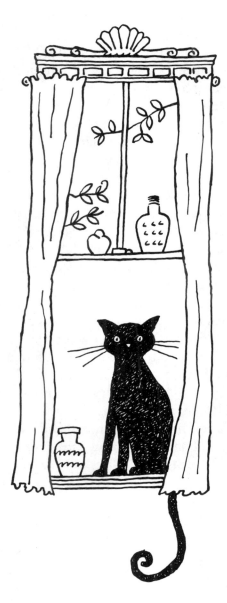

CHAPTER 1

What is Menopause?

The word *menopause* means different things to different women. For some, menopause is a process that begins at mid-life and lasts for the rest of their lives. Other women think of menopause as the symptoms, such as hot flashes and night sweats, that they go through around age 50 as their hormonal levels decrease. In reality, the word *menopause* refers to the end of all menstrual bleeding. While most women go through menopause between the ages of 48 and 52, some women cease menstruating as young as their late thirties or early forties, while others continue to menstruate into their mid-fifties.

For most women, the process that leads up to menopause occurs gradually, triggered by a slowdown in the function of their ovaries. This process begins four to six years before the last menstrual period and continues for several years after. During this time, there is a decrease in the estrogen production from the ovaries, finally dropping to such low levels that the periods become irregular and finally cease entirely. For some women this transition to a new hormonal equilibrium is easy and uneventful. For many women, however, the transition is difficult and fraught with many uncomfortable symptoms, such as hot flashes, night sweats, mood swings, and vaginal dryness. Some degree of symptoms is experienced by as many as 80 percent of all women going through menopause. To understand menopause better, let's look at the normal menstrual cycle to see what changes occur as women go toward menopause.

The Normal Menstrual Cycle

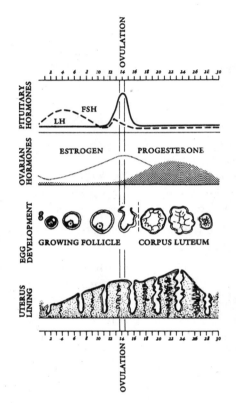

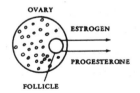

Each month women in their fertile years (before the ages of 45 to 50) go through menstruation, the shedding of the lining of the uterus. The lining of the uterus increases in thickness throughout the monthly cycle because of an increase in the blood supply and micronutrients. This thickening prepares the uterus for the growth and development of the fertilized egg, which will live in the uterus for the next nine months. If pregnancy does not occur, then this lining is not needed. The uterus cleanses itself of the cells with the monthly bleeding.

The eggs rest in an inactive form called follicles in the ovary each month. The ovaries are located in the woman's pelvic region and contain all the eggs she will ever have. At birth, each female has approximately one million eggs. Each month, hormones from the pituitary gland called FSH and LH cause the follicles to ripen and one of them to grow into an egg. In doing so, the follicle begins to produce the hormones estrogen and progesterone. Besides preparing the egg to be fertilized, these hormones also stimulate the lining of the uterus to prepare a proper home for the egg to grow. The estrogen and progesterone also control the obvious physical signs of femininity, such as breast development and growth of pubic hair. Estrogen increases during the first half of the cycle. Progesterone output occurs after midcycle when ovulation occurs. Ovulation is the production by one ovary of a mature egg cell, or ovarian follicle, which travels down the fallopian tube to the uterus and signals the time when a pregnancy can occur.

As a woman approaches menopause, the number of eggs in her ovaries begins to decrease. This decrease is progressive throughout life and is due to a built-in life-span, as well as a combination of environmental stress factors (like exposure to toxic chemicals and radiation, which can damage and destroy the eggs). By the time a woman reaches menopause, most of her eggs have been destroyed and the ovaries have ceased to function. The end result, by her fifties, is a marked decrease in estrogen and progesterone output. The next section will examine the symptoms that occur as a woman goes through the years leading up to and coinciding with the time of menopause.

Irregular Heavy Bleeding

The decrease in ovulation and hormonal output that occurs in the middle to late forties may cause irregular heavy bleeding in many women. The menstrual cycle may shorten, with the periods coming closer together. Bleeding may also be extremely heavy and may extend for a longer time. A one-week to ten-day menstrual period is not unusual, with some women bleeding throughout the entire month. This blood loss can be dangerous, since it can lead to anemia. As the time of menopause approaches, the pattern reverses, with the periods become farther apart and the flow scantier. The heavy bleeding phase can be treated with an operation called a dilatation and curettage (D&C).

The D&C will stop the bleeding and can also rule out other causes of bleeding, such as cancer. With this procedure, the lining of the uterus is removed by a suction or scraping technique while the patient is under local or total anesthesia. The cells are then analyzed for any abnormal patterns. If the bleeding problem is due to the hormonal imbalances leading up to menopause, the symptoms may recur. In this case, the bleeding may be treated with progestins—hormone supplements, similar to your natural progesterone. Natural progesterone acts to limit the amount of bleeding from the lining of your uterus during the second half of your menstrual cycle. Premenopausal women are deficient in progesterone, and may use progestin to limit the bleeding. Progestins can be taken during the same period (for one to two weeks at the end of your cycle). When they are stopped, you will have a bleeding episode, similar to a normal period, which lasts less than a week. Many environmental factors, such as emotional stress, cigarette smoking, and excessive alcohol intake can worsen the bleeding problem. All of these factors can make you more susceptible to heavy irregu-

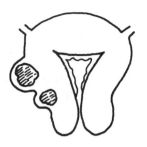

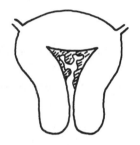

lar bleeding because of their negative effects. Techniques to deal with these problems are given in the Self Help section of this book. Medical studies have shown that deficiencies of iron, vitamin C, and bioflavonoids can worsen or even cause heavy irregular menstrual bleeding. Adequate amounts of these nutrients should be included in your diet and as supplements.

While most cases of irregular heavy bleeding are due to your fluctuating hormonal levels as you go toward menopause, other medical problems can cause bleeding, too. These include fibroid tumors (an overgrowth in the muscular tissue of the uterus), polyps, uterine cancer, and cervical cancer. For these reasons, any serious bleeding problems should be evaluated by your own doctor. While these problems are relatively uncommon compared to irregular bleeding because of hormonal imbalance, they should be diagnosed early while they are still easy to cure.

Hot Flashes

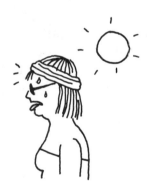

Hot flashes are one of the most uncomfortable symptoms that menopausal women complain about. They are sudden and intense episodes of warmth and heat that women experience around and after the time of menopause. These episodes come on unexpectedly, with a woman suddenly noticing that she feels warm and may need to remove a sweater or jacket. This is often accompanied by varying amounts of sweating, mild in some women and profuse in others. After the initial period of warmth, the sweating cools down her skin temperature and causes her to shiver. This temperature instability may be very uncomfortable for many women, causing them to alternately shed or add clothes. Hot flashes often begin on the chest, neck, or face, and radiate to other parts of the body. Eighty percent of women in menopause experience hot flashes, with forty percent of these women having symptoms severe enough to seek medical care. While most hot flashes appear to occur without any specific environmental trigger, it has been observed that coffee and alcohol intake may cause a flash to occur. The frequency, intensity, and duration of hot flashes vary greatly. For most women they last for two to three minutes, but they can

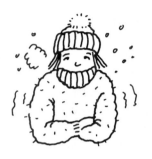

last longer, even up to an hour in some cases. In the majority of women, the symptoms begin to subside within four to six years after the last menstrual period.

The cause of the hot flash is unclear, but it appears to be related to the decrease in estrogen output at the time of menopause. The pituitary gland responds to the drop in ovarian hormones by increasing its level of gonadotrophins in an effort to elevate estrogen levels. The pituitary, in turn, is stimulated by releasing factors from the hypothalamus, which also regulates temperature control. Thus, the "thermostat" in the brain is affected by the pituitary gland and by ovarian hormonal instability. The most common medical treatment for this problem is estrogen replacement therapy. This is usually quite effective in stopping the hot flashes. It is not curative, however, and hot flashes can recur if the estrogen is stopped. It is important that a woman experiencing hot flashes keep cool. Plenty of cool water throughout the day, small meals, and avoidance of alcohol help to keep the body temperature down. It is also important not to overheat your house or overdress. Emotional upset can also worsen hot flashes, so calming techniques such as meditation and deep breathing may also be helpful. Medical research also suggests that supplementation with vitamin E and bioflavonoids may help control hot flashes. There have also been medical studies on a number of naturally occurring plant sources of estrogen. These and other strategies for dealing with hot flashes are discussed in more detail in the Self Help section of this book.

Vaginal and Urinary Tract Changes

As estrogen levels decrease with the onset of menopause, the tissues of the vagina and urethra undergo a number of changes. The vaginal and urethral linings become thinner, drier, and inelastic. There is a decrease in the blood supply to the vaginal and urethral area. The cervix secretes much less mucous than in a woman's fertile years. The vagina actually shrinks and becomes much shorter and narrower at the opening.

What does this mean in terms of a woman's lifestyle during the menopause years? Sexual intercourse often becomes much more

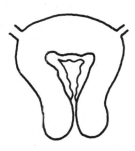

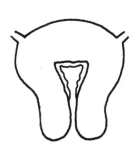

painful and uncomfortable. Sexual arousal no longer causes the same level of lubrication, and the capacity for vaginal expansion in response to sexual arousal may decrease. Vaginal infections may become more frequent because the tissues are easily traumatized. The changes that occur in the urethral tissues may increase the frequency of urination. Women find that they have to get up at night to void. Even more frustrating for some women is the tendency to leak urine when they laugh, sneeze, or cough.

Luckily, there are many methods to help relieve the vaginal and urethral changes. Estrogen can be taken in pill form or applied as a cream to the vaginal tissues on a regular basis. (Testosterone cream also may be used.) These treatments are very effective in thickening and healing the vaginal and urethral tissues. Unfortunately, even with estrogen therapy, the woman does not lubricate as effectively with sexual arousal. An additional lubricant like KY jelly can be very helpful in solving this problem. Regular orgasm and tender, sensitive lovemaking can help to relax the pelvic muscles and improve blood flow to the vaginal tissues. Supplementation with vitamins and herbs may also be helpful.

Vitamin E has been used to aid in the treatment of atrophic vaginitis. Vitamins E and A have also been used successfully to treat vulvovaginitis and vulvar leukoplakia, a skin condition generally experienced after menopause. A variety of herbs such as cohosh and licorice have been found to have estrogenic activity and may also be useful in treating these symptoms.

Psychological Symptoms of Menopause

Women may note mild to marked changes in their moods during the time of menopause. These symptoms include insomnia (often associated with hot flashes), irritability, anxiety, and depression. The physical instability due to the fluctuation in estrogen and progesterone as they readjust to a new and lower level of equilibrium can be mirrored by emotional changes, too. Both estrogen and progesterone have been studied for their effects on mood: if estrogen predominates, women tend to feel anxious; if pregesterone predominates, women may feel depressed. With a decrease in both hormones, symptoms can run the gamut from irritability to depression.

These mood changes are seen not only in menopause but also in a variety of other conditions marked by hormonal imbalances, including premenstrual syndrome, depression following childbirth or following surgical removal of the ovaries, and as side effects of the birth control pill. The severity of the symptoms is probably due to the woman's individual biochemistry, as well as to social factors. Women have worse symptoms if they are under severe emotional stress or have aggravating dietary habits such as excessive caffeine, sugar, or alcohol intake.

There are many treatments that can help women enjoy a calmer and more peaceful state of mind during the menopause years. Many studies of hormonal replacement therapy show beneficial effects on the psychological symptoms with various regimens of estrogen, progesterone, and androgens in menopausal women. For women who don't want to use hormonal therapy, there are other helpful treatments, including the use of tryptophan (an amino acid that has a calming effect) and mild herbal teas, such as camomile and valerian root, taken at bedtime. Regular exercise can improve one's mood tremendously, as can meditation and other relaxation techniques. Supplementation with such appropriate nutrients as potassium, magnesium, vitamins B, E, and bioflavonoids can also help to decrease fatigue, anxiety, and depression, and can improve one's mood and well-being.

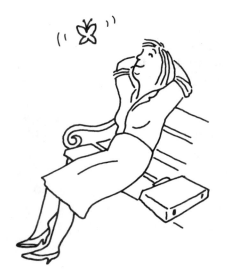

Osteoporosis

Osteoporosis is one of the most severe health problems that can occur in menopause. Both women and men tend to lose bone mass with age, and this process is accelerated in women with the onset of menopause. Estrogen has an important role in maintaining the structure and calcification of bone. With the drop in estrogen at menopause, this crucial hormonal support is withdrawn. In addition, with advancing age women may lose the ability to absorb and assimilate calcium from their diet. Because calcium is an important

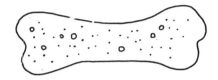

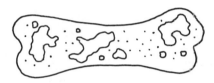

component of bone tissue, poor calcium absorption or an inadequate dietary supply can weaken bones.

There are many other genetic and lifestyle factors that can increase your risk of osteoporosis. These include a diet high in salt, protein, caffeine, or alcohol. Inadequate vitamin D levels (either from lack of sun exposure or low dietary intake) can affect your ability to absorb calcium. Women who smoke are at higher risk of osteoporosis, as are women who are short and thin. Exercise is necessary for bone strength and mass. Unfortunately, many women become more sedentary and housebound with age. A family history of female relatives with osteoporosis puts you at higher risk, as does a Northern European or ethnic background. (The exception are black women, who develop the disease less frequently.) All of these factors combine to put twenty-five percent of the female population at high risk for developing osteoporosis.

Although the degree of osteoporosis worsens significantly in a woman's fifties, the clinical signs and symptoms usually develop in the sixties and seventies. Fractures or compression of the vertebrae, and hip fractures are the most common results of osteoporosis. Compression of the vertebrae can cause a humped back, loss of height, or back pain. Hip fractures are equally common, with over a hundred thousand cases per year. One-third of these women die from complications, and many others suffer chronic disability due to injury.

It is important to treat osteoporosis with prevention rather than letting it develop into an advanced and disabling condition. Estrogen supplementation may help prevent osteoporosis in women who are at high risk for developing this problem. Daily weight-bearing exercise such as walking, climbing stairs, dancing, or slow jogging is a must. Bones respond to exercise by becoming stronger and thicker. Calcium and vitamin D supplementation should be started even in the forties, before menopause begins. Salt, protein, coffee, and alcohol should be replaced by a modified vegetarian diet high in fruits, vegetables, grains, legumes, herbs, and smaller portions of meat protein. All of these strategies and others to prevent osteoporosis are discussed in detail in the Self Help portion of this book.

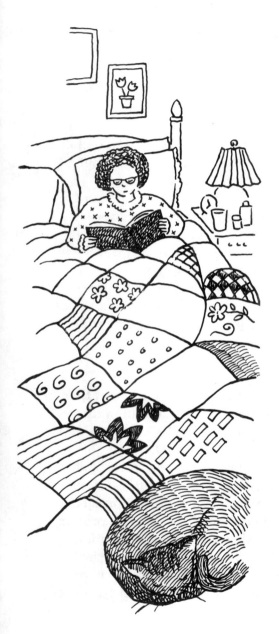

CHAPTER 2

Other Health Problems Beyond Menopause

This chapter presents a survey of other health problems as well as age-related changes that become more prevalent in women after the menopause years. The withdrawal of hormonal support that occurs with menopause seems to increase the frequency of many diseases. The visible effects of aging also increase after mid-life. For example, in many women there is an increase in wrinkling of the skin and thinning of the hair. Diseases of the female body, such as breast and uterine cancer, as well as low thyroid conditions, become more prevalent after menopause. Women show an acceleration in their development of cardiovascular disease and elevated blood pressure.

Read this chapter carefully to see if you are at high risk for any of these problems. Many of these diseases can be prevented or alleviated by attention to good preventive health care and a variety of self help techniques. Many of these techniques are presented in the Self Help section of this book.

Breast Cancer

Breast cancer is the most common cancer in women up to age 74. In 1985, 199,000 new cases of breast cancer were diagnosed, with 37,000 deaths. Most cases are diagnosed between 45 and 55 years of age, although nearly one-third occur in women over 65. It is estimated that one woman out of eleven will develop breast cancer during her lifetime. Although the causes of breast cancer are not known, a number of factors are associated with an increased risk of the disease, including:

- Previous breast cancer
- Close female relatives (mother, sister, grandmother, aunt) with breast cancer
- Atypical hyperplasia diagnosed on a breast biopsy
- Early menstruation (before age 12) and/or late menopause (after age 50)
- Childlessness or late motherhood (after age 35)
- Member of certain ethnic groups—e.g., European Jews, Northern Europeans
- High-fat diet
- Estrogen replacement therapy without progesterone
- Low levels of selenium
- Low levels of iodine

Early detection of the disease can have a significant effect on survival rates. This is particularly important for women in the high-risk group. Early methods of detection include:

- Complete monthly breast self-examination
- Annual breast exam by a physician
- Baseline mammogram between ages of 35 and 40
- Yearly mammogram after age 50 (every other year for women between 40 and 50 years and high-risk women over 35)

Current treatment options for diagnosed disease are considerably broader than a generation ago, when the Halsted radical mastectomy (complete removal of the breast, lymph nodes, and surrounding muscle) was the standard treatment. Current options include modified radical mastectomy, lumpectomy with removal of malignancy and a minimum of surrounding tissue, and simple mastectomy with radiation. Various combinations of surgery, chemotherapy, and radiation have had a significant effect on long-term survival with invasive disease. Attention to prevention,

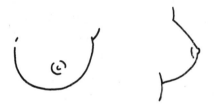

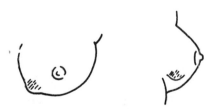

including maintenance of a low-fat diet, is important for women at high risk. Research studies suggest that supplemental selenium and iodine decrease the risk of breast cancer.

Hypothyroidism

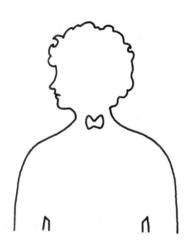

Hypothyroidism is far more common in females than in males. The disease becomes increasingly prevalent with age. Classic symptoms of hypothyroidism include hoarse voice, constipation, slowness of speech, thought, and movement, intolerance to cold, thickening and scaling of skin, facial puffiness, and delay of deep tendon reflexes. However, clinical diagnosis of hypothyroidism in older women may be difficult because many women do not have the typical symptoms. In many older women debilitation and apathy may be the only signs of low thyroid function. Medical studies suggest that thyroid screening in older patients should be a routine part of their physical examination.

Therapy in older women does not differ greatly from that of younger patients, except that older patients may require a much lower maintenance dose of thyroxine. Self help aspects of treatment and prevention include adequate iodine either in the diet or in supplementary form. There is also evidence that adequate intake of vitamins A, E, and iodine may be necessary to maintain thyroid health and integrity.

Cancer of the Cervix

After breast cancer, this is one of the most common cancers in women. Approximately 60,000 cases per year are diagnosed. Luckily, early detection with Pap smears allows three-quarters of the cases to be picked up in an early or noninvasive stage when a complete cure is possible. The incidence of cervical cancer increases with age, as the malignant process progresses through stages of cervical cell abnormality called dysplasia, then localized cancer, and finally invasive cancer (the most serious form). Risk factors include early sexual activity with multiple partners, herpes infection, and childbearing during teenage years. Cervical cancer grows

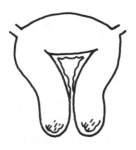

slowly, with localized cancer appearing ten to fifteen years earlier than invasive cancer. Because of the slow growth of most cervical cancers, women should be sure to get regular Pap smears to detect cancer at an early stage. Most women, however, do not have to have a Pap smear every year. If you have had three normal Pap smears, most doctors nowadays will recommend that you repeat every three years.

Medical studies suggest that supplementation with folic acid, vitamin C, and vitamin A can help prevent abnormal cellular patterns in the cervix. This supplementation may even help to prevent cervical cancer. If the cervical cell abnormalities are caught at the precancerous stage, the problem can be treated by freezing the cervix (cryotherapy) or surgical removal of part of the cervix. Once the changes become cancerous, however, the uterus must be removed. Early detection is crucial because the survival rate drops greatly once the disease spreads beyond the uterus.

Uterine Cancer

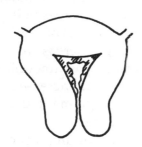

Uterine cancer is usually found in women after menopause. The incidence of this disease rises sharply in the sixties, though it can also be found in younger women (especially those on oral contraceptive pills). Excess estrogen in the body seems to increase your risk of developing this disease. Obese women are at particular risk because body fat converts androstenedione, an adrenal hormone, to estrone, a type of estrogen. Thus, the more body fat you have, the higher your level of estrogen in the menopause years. Women who take estrogen replacement therapy without progesterone multiply by five the risk of developing uterine cancer. Other risk factors include:

- Diabetes mellitus
- Early menstruation
- Childlessness
- Past history of breast cancer
- High blood pressure
- Low levels of selenium
- Low levels of iodine

Many women who develop uterine cancer may have abnormally heavy menstrual bleeding, although this is not always true. The disease can be diagnosed with a Pap smear or biopsy of the uterine lining. Both of these procedures can often be done at a doctor's office. Early detection is critical because total cure is still possible at this stage. Uterine cancer usually requires the removal of the uterus or a hysterectomy.

Women at high risk of uterine cancer should make a special effort to control their weight, follow a low-fat diet, and avoid excessive alcohol intake (alcohol can increase the level of estrogen in the body). They should also include adequate iodine and selenium in their diet, either in their food or as supplements.

The Skin at Menopause

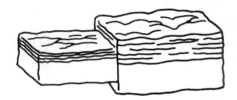

The loss of hormonal support at menopause causes changes in the structure and texture of the skin. With the decrease in both estrogen and androgen (the male hormone that all women make in small amounts), the skin becomes drier, thinner, and tends to secrete less oil. The loss of fat beneath the skin adds to the appearance of aging, since this diminishes the look of plumpness associated with youth. The loss of blood circulation to the skin causes the skin to lose its healthy pink color and to become increasingly pale with age. Other signs of skin's aging include the loss of tone and elasticity that results in wrinkling and sagging. There is an increased transparency of the skin that causes a parchmentlike appearance with age. After menopause there is an increased unevenness and roughness in both texture and pigmentation. Skin spots, lesions, and cancers increase after mid-life.

Many of these skin changes could be avoided or diminished if women would avoid sun exposure and cigarette smoking; both of these habits exact a terrible toll on the skin and cause an acceleration of skin's aging. Sun exposure is particularly dangerous because it damages both the skin and its underlying supportive layers, which worsens wrinkling and dryness. Women who overexpose their skin to the sun have much higher levels of skin cancer and precancerous lesions.

Women in the menopause years should wear adequate sunscreen (SPF 15 or more) when going outdoors. I also recommend mechanical barriers such as long-sleeve shirts and hats to avoid excessive sun exposure. Besides cigarette smoking, it is important to minimize alcohol intake, which can dehydrate the skin further. Women with dry skin should avoid excessive washing with soap and hot water, as this can further denude the skin of its protective oils. On the plus side, daily exercise is excellent because it improves blood circulation and nutrient flow to the skin. Medical research has shown that high levels of vitamins A and E have extremely beneficial effects on clearing up skin diseases, and they promote healthy skin generally. Supplementation should be considered as well as adequate sources of vitamins A and E in your diet. Good food sources include carrots, squash, peppers, leafy green vegetables, yams, and vegetable oils.

Cardiovascular Disease

This represents the most common cause of death in women by the time of menopause. By age 55, a woman is more likely to die from cardiovascular disease than from any other cause. For women between the ages of 55 and 64, there are 280 heart attack deaths per 100,000 population; after age 65, this increases to 2,001 deaths per 100,000. Women at high risk for cardiovascular disease also have a higher risk of stroke and hypertension. Risk factors include:

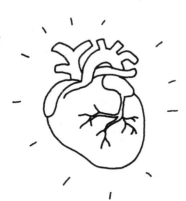

- Strong family history of cardiovascular disease (parents, sibling), especially before age 60
- Cigarette habit
- Diabetes
- Elevated serum cholesterol and serum triglycerides
- Elevated blood pressure
- Use of oral contraceptives past the age of 35
- Lack of exercise
- Obesity

There is evidence from the Framingham Study (a medical study ongoing since 1949), as well as many other medical studies, that modification of these risk factors may have an effect on morbidity and mortality. There has been an encouraging decline in cardiovascular mortality in the United States, particularly in stroke and coronary mortality in the seventh and eighth decades of life. Ideally, multiple preventive measures should be instituted as early in life as possible, but even late in life some measures may be helpful. Nutrients that may play a useful role in managing cardiovascular disease and hypertension include potassium, calcium, manganese, magnesium, and vitamins E, C, and niacin.

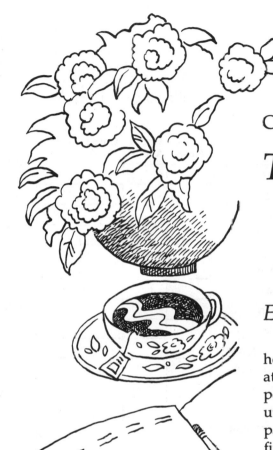

CHAPTER 3

The Menopause Workbook

Evaluating Your Symptoms

The Workbook section will help you to evaluate your habits and how they may contribute to menopause symptoms, and to evaluate your risk of developing menopause-related problems like osteoporosis, as well as such female health problems as breast and uterine cancer. These problems become more common after menopause. If you take the time to fill out the evaluation sheets, you'll find it easier to recognize your weak areas, and you can put together your own treatment program from the following chapters for the best menopause relief.

First, fill out the lifestyle habit evaluations. They will help you assess specific areas of your life to see which of your habit patterns are contributing to your menopause symptoms. Next, fill out the evaluation of risk factors for female health problems. This will show you if you are at risk for a particular disease. Working with the preventive health care techniques in the rest of the book can help improve your health and lessen your risks.

When you have completed the evaluations, you will be ready to go on to the next chapter and begin your treatment program.

Lifestyle Habits and Menopause

Eating Habits and Menopause

Check off the number of times you eat the following foods:

Foods	Never	Once a Month	Once a Week	Twice a Week Plus
coffee				X
black tea			X	
soft drinks	X			X
cow's milk			X	X
cow's cheese			X	X
butter				X
yogurt	X		X	
eggs			X	
chocolate			X	
sugar	·			
alcohol	X			
beef	X			
pork	X			
lamb	X			
white bread			X	
white noodles			X	
white flour pastries	X			
added salt				X
bouillon	X			
commercial salad dressing	X			
catsup	X			
hot dogs	X			
bologna	X			
salami	X			

Foods	Never	Once a Month	Once a Week	Twice a Week Plus
avocado				
beans				
beets				
broccoli				
brussels sprouts				
cabbage				
carrots				
celery				
collard greens				
cucumbers				
eggplant				
garlic				
horseradish				
kale				
lettuce				
mustard greens				
okra				
onions				
parsnips				
peas				
potatoes				
radishes				
rutabagas				
spinach				
squash				

Foods	Never	Once a Month	Once a Week	Twice a Week Plus
tomatoes				
turnips				
turnip greens				
yams				
almonds				
filberts				
peanuts				
pecans				
walnuts				
barley				
brown rice				
buckwheat				
corn				
millet				
oatmeal				
pumpkin seeds				
rye				
sesame seeds				
sunflower seeds				

Foods	Never	Once a Month	Once a Week	Twice a Week Plus
apples				
apricots				
bananas				
berries				
grapefruit				
grapes				
melons				
peaches				
oranges				
papayas				
pears				
pineapples				
seasonal fruits				
corn oil				
olive oil				
sesame oil				
safflower oil				
fish				
poultry				

Key to eating habits and menopause. All the foods in the shaded area are high-stress foods that can worsen your menopause symptoms. If you eat a significant number of these foods, or if you eat any of these foods frequently, your nutritional habits may be contributing significantly to your symptoms, and you can probably benefit greatly from the dietary guidelines in the nutritional chapters.

All the foods from avocado to poultry are high-nutrient, low-stress foods that may help to relieve or prevent menopause symptoms and should be included frequently in your diet. If you are already eating many of these foods and few of the high-stress foods, chances are your nutritional habits are good, and nutrition may not be a significant factor in reducing your menopause symptoms. The other self-help techniques, such as stress reduction and exercise, may be more important to you.

How Menopause Stress Affects Your Body

Check the places where tension most commonly localizes in your body:

☐ Shoulders ☐ Headache
☐ Neck and throat ☐ Eyestrain
☐ Grinding teeth ☐ Arms
☐ Lower back ☐ Stomach muscles

Key to what stress does to your body. This evaluation should help you become aware of where you store stress in your body. Everyone has her own particular area. This accumulation increases your general level of fatigue and lowers your energy.

Try to remain aware of the areas where you store tension. When you feel tension building up in them, do the stretches and stress reduction exercises described in the book—often they will help reduce the tension significantly.

Menopause Stress Symptoms

Check how often you are affected by the following:

	Never	Mild	Moderate	Severe
insomnia				
irritability				
anxiety				
anger				
feeling constantly stressed				
nervous tension				
mood swings				
fatigue				
depression				
hopelessness				
low self-esteem				

Key to menopause stress symptoms. Many women during mid-life and beyond notice a change in their emotional state with the decrease in hormones that occurs at menopause. Some women complain of anxiety, irritability, and insomnia, while others suffer more from fatigue and depression. If you have any of these symptoms, look at the many self help treatment options described in this book. Try several of them and see which ones make you feel the best.

Exercise Habits and Menopause

Check off the number of times you do any of the following:

	Never	Once a Month	Once or Twice a Week	3 Times a Week or more
fast walking				
running				
swimming				
bicycling				
tennis				
aerobic dancing				
yoga				
squash				
racquetball				
golf				
weight lifting				
martial arts				
bowling				
square dancing				
ballroom dancing				

Key to exercise habits and menopause. Regular exercise is absolutely necessary for women during the menopause years and beyond. Besides improving circulation to the pelvic organs, it also helps to preserve bone mass and strength. It is vitally important for cardio-vascular health and fitness. Exercise is also a good outlet for menopause-related stress. If your total number of exercise periods per week is less than three, they should be increased and the chapters on various kinds of exercise for menopause will be important to you.

If you are exercising more than three times a week, keep doing your exercises; they are improving your health and well-being. You may want to add specific corrective exercises from this book to your present regime. Choose them to fit your individual symptoms from the Complete Treatment Chart on pages 32–35.

Osteoporosis

Osteoporosis affects 25 percent of all American women by the age of 80. It is a significant cause of injury and death in older women. It is very important that you read the risk factors listed below and work to correct any that you might have. Osteoporosis can be effectively prevented with adequate exercise, calcium and vitamin D intake, and with proper dietary habits.

RISK FACTORS	YES	NO
Member of a non-black ethnic group	☐	☐
Female relatives with osteoporosis	☐	☐
Early menopause (before age 40)	☐	☐
Being short and thin	☐	☐
Childlessness	☐	☐
High alcohol use	☐	☐
High caffeine use	☐	☐
Smoking	☐	☐
Low-calcium diet	☐	☐
Lack of vitamin D	☐	☐
High-salt diet	☐	☐
High-protein diet	☐	☐
Chronic diarrhea or surgical removal of stomach or small intestine	☐	☐
Daily use of cortisone	☐	☐
Use of thyroid medication (over 2 grains), Dilantin, or aluminum-containing antacids	☐	☐

Breast Cancer

You may have a higher risk of breast cancer if any of the following risk factors are positive. I recommend that you follow the nutritional guidelines and exercise techniques for breast health in the Self Help section of this book. It is important that you do regular breast self-examinations. Consult your doctor if you discover a breast lump or have any other symptom that might indicate breast disease.

RISK FACTORS	YES	NO
Previous breast cancer	☐	☐
Close female relatives (mother, sister, grandmother, aunts) with breast cancer	☐	☐
Atypical hyperplasia (abnormal tissue pattern) diagnosed on a breast biopsy	☐	☐
Early menstruation (before age 12) and/or late menopause (after age 50)	☐	☐
Childlessness or late motherhood (after age 35)	☐	☐
Member of certain ethnic groups—e.g., European Jews, Northern Europeans	☐	☐
High-fat consumption in diet	☐	☐
Menopausal women using estrogen replacement therapy without progesterone	☐	☐
Low levels of selenium	☐	☐
Low levels of iodine	☐	☐
Frequent high-dose x-ray exposure of the breasts	☐	☐

Uterine Cancer

You are at higher risk of uterine cancer if you have any of the risk factors listed below. Be sure to follow the nutritional and other self-help techniques for uterine health. Get regular Pap smears and see your doctor if you have any abnormal vaginal bleeding after menopause, as this can be a sign of uterine cancer.

RISK FACTORS	YES	NO
Women past the age of 65	☐	☐
Menopausal women using estrogen replacement therapy without progesterone	☐	☐
Obesity	☐	☐
Diabetes mellitus	☐	☐
Early menstruation	☐	☐
Childlessness	☐	☐
Past history of breast cancer	☐	☐
High blood pressure	☐	☐
Low levels of selenium	☐	☐
Low levels of iodine	☐	☐

Cancer of the Cervix

You are at higher risk of cervical cancer if you have any of the risk factors listed below. Cervical cancer is easy to detect on a Pap smear. You should have a Pap smear done on a regular basis if you are at high risk for cervical cancer. Be sure to follow the recommendations in the self help chapters of the book.

RISK FACTORS	YES	NO
Women past the age of 45	☐	☐
Early sexual activity	☐	☐
Multiple sexual partners	☐	☐
Childbearing during teenage years	☐	☐
History of venereal warts	☐	☐
History of genital herpes infection	☐	☐
Low dietary vitamin A intake	☐	☐
Low dietary vitamin C intake	☐	☐
Low dietary folic acid intake	☐	☐

Hypothyroidism

Hypothyroidism increases with age and is far more common in women than in men. If you have any of the risk factors listed below, you may be hypothyroid. This can be easily diagnosed by blood testing. Follow the recommendations in the self help chapters for optimal thyroid health.

SYMPTOMS	YES	NO
Hoarse voice	☐	☐
Constipation	☐	☐
Slowness of speech, thought, and movement	☐	☐
Fatigue	☐	☐
Intolerance to cold	☐	☐
Thickening and scaling of your skin	☐	☐
Facial puffiness	☐	☐
Delay of deep tendon reflexes	☐	☐
Low dietary iodine	☐	☐
Axillary (armpit) temperature below 97.8°F	☐	☐
Elevated cholesterol	☐	☐

Cardiovascular Disease

Women's risk of cardiovascular disease increases dramatically after menopause. This risk can be effectively decreased with proper attention to a variety of lifestyle factors, including nutrition, exercise, and stress reduction. If you are at high risk of developing cardiovascular disease, follow the self help strategies in this book. You may also want to see your doctor for further evaluation.

RISK FACTORS INCLUDE:	YES	NO
Strong family history of cardiovascular disease (parents, siblings), especially before age 60	☐	☐
Cigarette habit	☐	☐
Diabetes mellitus	☐	☐
Elevated serum triglycerides	☐	☐
Elevated serum cholesterol	☐	☐
Use of oral contraceptives past the age of 35	☐	☐
Obesity	☐	☐
Elevated blood pressure	☐	☐
High level of emotional stress	☐	☐
Lack of exercise (sedentary lifestyle)	☐	☐
High alcohol intake	☐	☐

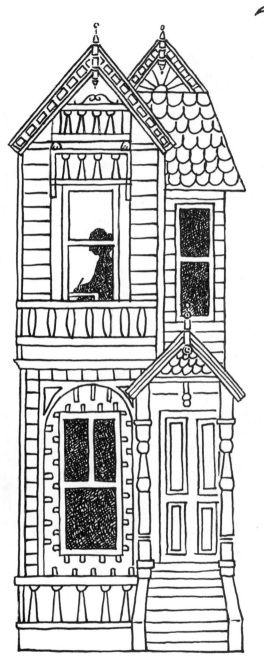

CHAPTER 4

The Menopause Self Help Program

Now that you know all about the causes and symptoms of menopause, you are ready to begin your treatment program. This program is set up so that you can individualize a treatment plan for yourself. The methods that you need are contained in the chapters that follow. These include diet, nutrition, stress reduction, exercise, acupressure massage, pressure point exercises, and yoga.

This chapter contains a master plan that will help you to put your own program together. The chart on the next pages will tell you which treatments to use for your symptoms.

There are two basic ways to use the treatment plan. You can find your symptoms in the chart and turn directly to the treatments for those symptoms. What will work for you can be found easily if you try all the therapies listed under your symptoms. You will probably find that some make you feel better than others. Establish the regimen that works for you and use it each month. Or you can read straight through the rest of the book, get a general overview of the various approaches, and find those you are interested in trying. You can then use the treatment chart for quick spot work and a large overview. Whichever way you choose, if you follow your own plan faithfully, you will begin to see improvements in your symptoms and your life very quickly—within a month or two.

MENOPAUSE TREATMENT CHART

	General Health, Fitness and Flexibility	Entire Female Reproductive Tract	Irregular Heavy Bleeding (Menorrhagia)	Hot Flashes	Atrophic Vaginitis	Sexual Desire, Frigidity
Medication			Progestins	Estrogen	Estrogen Topical Creme	
Nutrition	The Menopause Self Help Diet	The Menopause Self Help Diet	The Menopause Self Help Diet	The Menopause Self Help Diet	The Menopause Self Help Diet	The Menopause Self Help Diet
Vitamins	Vitamin and Mineral Formula, page 114	Vitamin and Mineral Formula, page 114	Vitamin and Mineral Formula, page 114; Emphasize Vitamin A, Bioflavonoids, Vitamin C, Iron	Vitamin and Mineral Formula, page 114; Emphasize Bioflavonoids, Vitamin E	Vitamin and Mineral Formula, page 114; Emphasize Bioflavonoids, Vitamin E	Vitamin and Mineral Formula, page 114
Herbs			Shepherd's Purse, Hawthorn Berry, Cherry, Grape Skin, Bilberry, Red Clover	Dong Quai, Black Cohosh, Blue Cohosh, Unicorn Root, False Unicorn Root, Fennel, Sarsaparilla, Red Clover, Wild Yam Root, Yam		

Lower Urinary Tract Changes	Psychological Symptoms of Menopause: Anxiety, Irritability, Insomnia	Psychological Symptoms of Menopause: Depression, Fatigue	Osteoporosis	Breast Disease	Thyroid Problems	Pelvic Disease: Uterus, Ovaries, Cervix
Estrogen	Tranquilizers	Anti-depressants	Estrogen and Progesterone	Medication Depends on Specific Disease	Thyroid Replacement Therapy	Medication Depends on Type of Disease
The Menopause Self Help Diet	The Menopause Self Help Diet	The Menopause Self Help Diet	The Menopause Self Help Diet	The Menopause Self Help Diet	The Menopause Self Help Diet	The Menopause Self Help Diet
Vitamin and Mineral Formula, page 114	Vitamin and Mineral Formula, page 114; Emphasize Vitamin B Complex, Magnesium	Vitamin and Mineral Formula, page 114; Emphasize Potassium, Magnesium, Vitamin B_{12}	Vitamin and Mineral Formula, page 114; Emphasize Calcium, Magnesium, Vitamin D, Zinc, Folic Acid	Vitamin and Mineral Formula, page 114; Emphasize Vitamin A, Vitamin E, Iodine, Selenium	Vitamin and Mineral Formula, page 114; Emphasize Iodine	Vitamin and Mineral Formula, page 114; Emphasize Vitamin A, Folic Acid, Vitamin C, Vitamin B_6
Coleus Forskohlii (pain), Goldenseal (infections), Uva Ursi (infections), Blackberry Root (infections), Wintergreen	Valerian Root, Passionflower, Peppermint, Catnip, Camomile, Hops	Oat Straw, Ginger, Cayenne Pepper, Dandelion Root, Siberian Ginseng, Blessed Thistle	Red Raspberry Leaf, Comfrey	Alfalfa, Kelp, Poke Root Poultices	Irish Moss, Kelp, Dulse, Sarsaparilla	

	General Health, Fitness and Flexibility	Entire Female Reproductive Tract	Irregular Heavy Bleeding (Menorrhagia)	Hot Flashes	Atrophic Vaginitis	Sexual Desire, Frigidity
General Exercises for Fitness and Flexibility	Exercises 1,2,3					
Stress Reduction	Menopause Stress Reduction Exercises	Menopause Stress Reduction Exercises	Menopause Stress Reduction Exercises	Menopause Stress Reduction Exercises	Menopause Stress Reduction Exercises	Menopause Stress Reduction Exercises
Acupressure Massage	Acupressure Exercise 1	Acupressure Exercises 1,2,3	Acupressure Exercises 2,3,4	Acupressure Exercises 2,6,7	Acupressure Exercises 2,3,8,9	Acupressure Exercises 2,10
Neurolymphatic Massage Points		NL-1,2		NL-1,2	NL-1,2	NL-1,2
Neurovascular Holding Points						
Yoga		Pump, Spinal Flex, Locust, Wide-Angle Pose, Upward Facing Dog		Pump, Spinal Flex, Locust, Wide-Angle Pose, Plow, Upward Facing Dog	Pump, Spinal Flex, Locust, Wide-Angle Pose, Upward Facing Dog	Pump, Spinal Flex, Locust, Wide-Angle Pose, Upward Facing Dog

Lower Urinary Tract Changes	Psychological Symptoms of Menopause: Anxiety, Irritability, Insomnia	Psychological Symptoms of Menopause: Depression, Fatigue	Osteoporosis	Breast Disease	Thyroid Problems	Pelvic Disease: Uterus, Ovaries, Cervix
Menopause Stress Reduction Exercises	Menopause Stress Reduction Exercises	Menopause Stress Reduction Exercises	Menopause Stress Reduction Exercises	Menopause Stress Reduction Exercises	Menopause Stress Reduction Exercises	Menopause Stress Reduction Exercises
Acupressure Exercises 2,3,10,11	Acupressure Exercises 1,12	Acupressure Exercise 13	Acupressure Exercise 14	Acupressure Exercise 15	Acupressure Exercises 5,13	Acupressure Exercises 2,3
NL-3,4	NL-5	NL-6		NL-7	NL-5	NL-1,2
	NV-1	NV-2				
Pump, Spinal Flex, Locust, Wide-Angle Pose, Upward Facing Dog	Pump, Sponge, Child's Pose	Upward Facing Dog, Bow	Pump, Spinal Flex, Wide-Angle Pose, Plow, Bow, Upward Facing Dog, Chest Expander, Lion, Tree	Upward Facing Dog, Chest Expander	Locust, Plow, Lion	Pump, Spinal Flex, Locust, Wide-Angle Pose, Upward Facing Dog

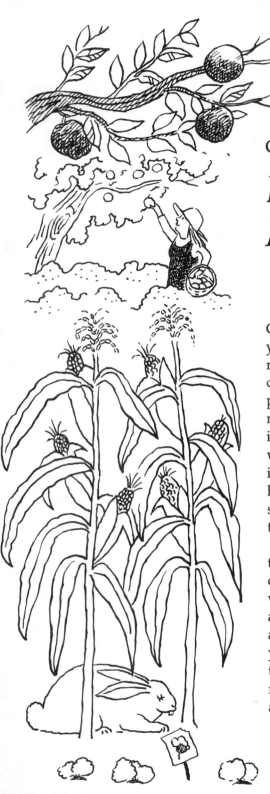

CHAPTER 5

Basic Principles of the Menopause Self Help Diet

Good nutrition is absolutely essential for women in the menopause years. The woman's body at mid-life is going through changes related to the aging process. All the body systems are slowing down and becoming less efficient and effective. Our digestive tract produces fewer enzymes and hydrochloric acid as we age, which makes digestion more difficult. The loss of hormonal support during menopause can adversely affect all systems of the body. Many women may notice that they tire more easily after menopause. The incidence of many common diseases like cancer, diabetes, and heart disease begins to rise sharply. Our diet, if it is full of high-stress foods like sugar, fat, alcohol, and caffeine, can accelerate these health problems related to the aging process.

A healthful and well-chosen diet is crucial if you want to maintain optimal health and go through the second half of your life disease-free, full of vigor and vitality. A well-chosen diet for women at mid-life includes fruits, vegetables, grains, beans, seeds and nuts, vegetable oils, and small amounts of lean meat, poultry, and fish. These foods will provide the important nutrients that your body needs to stay healthy and rebuild and repair any injury that it sustains. Many menopause problems—such as osteoporosis, hot flashes, and vaginal changes—can even be prevented and controlled by the right nutrition. Optimal food selection is one of the most important facts that you need to work with in your self-help program. This chapter gives you reliable information about the foods to eat during the menopause years, and which foods to avoid.

Foods for Menopause

The Women's Diet is a return to the whole fresh foods to which our bodies adapted over thousands of years. It emphasizes foods made from whole grains, legumes, vegetables, fruits, seeds and nuts, lean meats, fish, poultry, and oils.

Whole Grains

Whole grains include corn, barley, oats, rye, millet, buckwheat, brown rice, and wild rice. These are complex carbohydrates capable of stabilizing your blood sugar and helping tremendously to eliminate sugar craving. They are helpful in preventing or controlling diabetes mellitus, a dangerous disease which predisposes people toward heart disease, blood vessel problems, infections, and blindness. Fifty percent of our population above 60 have blood sugar abnormalities, due in great part to the tremendous amount of highly sugared foods and sweets Americans eat. Whole grains, with their natural sweetness, can satisfy much of this craving in a healthful way.

Grains are high in fiber, which is the indigestible part of plant food. The fiber in grain is very helpful in relieving constipation, as well as in preventing other diseases of the digestive tract such as diverticulitis and hiatus hernia. They may also have a protective effect against developing colon cancer, a disease found more commonly in people who eat a high-fat diet. Breast cancer and ovarian cancer are also found more frequently in persons eating a high-fat diet, particularly dairy products. Grains, with their low fat content, may have a protective effect against developing these diseases, too. When combined with beans, they are an excellent source of protein. They are highly nutritious and contain vitamins B, E, and various minerals. The whole grain or whole grain flour should be eaten instead of the refined flour product, because whole grain contains the nutrients and fiber.

Whole grains or whole grain flour can be prepared in a variety of ways, including whole grain cereals, bread, crackers, pancakes, waffles, and pasta. For many women I recommend emphasizing all grains except whole wheat. This is because wheat is highly allergenic and in many women can cause bloating and digestive problems. Luckily, there is a large range of non-wheat grain products available.

Whole-Grain Cereals. Your best bet if you shop in a local supermarket is the slow-cooking Quaker Oats (the quick-cooking kind is a refined grain product and should be avoided). Health food stores offer a larger choice of cereals. Puffed millet, puffed corn, and puffed rice are all available as cold breakfast cereals. Unsweetened granola, cream of rye, and buckwheat groats are also good.

Whole-Grain Bread. Take advantage of the many different whole-grain breads that are available at health food stores today—rice, sesame-millet, oatmeal, soy-potato, rye, and lima bean bread, among others. Choose brands without added sugar.

Crackers. Crackers can be used for snacks or open-face sandwiches. Brown rice cakes are particularly good when spread with soy spreads, tuna salad, or fruit and nut spreads.

Pancakes and Waffles. Pancakes and waffles can be made with buckwheat, rice flour, or triticale. Concentrated forms of sweeteners such as maple syrup, honey, and applesauce can be used in small amounts. See the Cookbook section for several delicious recipes.

Pasta. Pasta made out of buckwheat, rice, corn, and soy are readily available in health food and ethnic food stores. They are much more nutritious than refined wheat noodles and spaghetti. Whole grain pasta is also made with several delicately flavored vegetables, including artichokes and spinach.

Legumes

Legumes refer to the many members of the bean and pea family, some of the more common of which include lentils, kidney beans, pinto beans, mung beans, garbanzo beans, adzuki beans, and green peas. The many other members of the legume family can be used in many ways: they can become bases for thick soups, or they can be eaten in salads, or used in dips and casseroles. When eaten with grains they form a complete protein comparable to that in eggs or meat.

Legumes are very high in protein and when combined with grains they are an excellent complete source of amino acids. When served this way they are as high in quality protein as meat and eggs. For example, beans and rice or cornbread and split pea soup provide all the protein you need at a meal. Beans are also high in fiber and digest slowly. As with grains, their slow absorption from the digestive tract helps to regulate the blood sugar, and beans are an excellent food for women with diabetes or blood sugar imbalances. Some women do complain of gas when eating beans; this discomfort can be minimized by cooking them thoroughly and eating them in small amounts.

Vegetables

Most vegetables are extremely rich in vitamins and minerals. Vegetables high in vitamin A can be recognized by their yellow, orange, red, and dark green color. These include squash, sweet potatoes, peppers, carrots, kale and lettuce, as well as many other common foods. These foods should figure prominently in your diet because research shows that vitamin A can protect against cancer and immune deficiency. Of particular interest to menopausal women are the studies showing that vitamin A may protect against breast disease and cancer of the cervix. It is also necessary for healthy skin and eyes. Interestingly enough, vitamin A can be toxic when taken as a vitamin supplement because it is usually derived from sources like fish liver oil, which is fat soluble and can be toxic to the liver in doses above of 20,000 I.U. per day. The vitamin A found in vegetables is water soluble, is quite safe, and can be eaten in large amounts.

Many vegetables are also high in vitamin C, which has a protective effect against cancer and immune system problems. Vitamin C is particularly important for menopausal women since, along with iron and bioflavonoids, it can protect against excessive menstrual bleeding, a common problem as women approach menopause. It also seems to protect women from developing cervical cancer. Vegetables high in vitamin C include potatoes, peppers, peas, tomatoes, broccoli, brussels sprouts, cabbage, cauliflower, kale, and parsley. Vitamin C is also important for wound healing and healthy skin.

Vegetables contain many other important nutrients like iron, magnesium, and calcium. Leafy green vegetables like beet greens, collard, and dandelion greens are good sources of these important nutrients that protect against osteoporosis and excessive menstrual bleeding. Onions and garlic decrease the blood's clotting tendency and lower serum cholesterol, which can help decrease the incidence of stroke and heart attack. Studies indicate that mushrooms may have a similar effect and may stimulate immune function. Some vegetables such as kelp are high in iodine and trace minerals, which are essential for healthy thyroid function. Use kelp as a seasoning to sprinkle on vegetables and grains.

Eat your vegetables raw or lightly steamed to preserve their nutrient value. Do not boil or overcook, as vitamins and minerals can be lost through improper preparation. The following chapter contains important information on the best ways to prepare vegetables, as well as many simple and delicious recipes.

Fruits

Fruits are the source of many excellent nutrients, including a wide range of vitamins and minerals. Fruits tend to be very high in potassium, which helps to lower high blood pressure and protects against heart disease. Potassium also decreases bloat and fluid retention. Medical studies show that potassium is helpful in reducing menopause-related fatigue. Fruits high in potassium include bananas, oranges, grapefruits, berries, peaches, apricots, and melons. Fruits are an excellent source of vitamin C, which provides important protection against cancer and infectious disease. Most whole fruits contain some vitamin C; berries, oranges, and melons provide exceptionally high levels of this essential nutrient. Orange and yellow fruits like papaya, persimmon, apricot, and tangerine should be included in your diet because of their high vitamin A levels.

The delicious sweet flavors of fruits make them a healthy substitute for candies, cookies, cakes, and other highly sugared foods. Use them as a snack or dessert instead of ice cream or pastry. While fruit is high in sugar, the high fiber helps to slow down digestion, curb your appetite, and stabilize your blood sugar level. Fruit is also an excellent food for women who tend to be constipated; pineapple and papaya are excellent fruits for regulating bowel function and improving digestion. They contain enzymes that help to digest proteins and speed up bowel transit time. Be careful, however, not to drink too much fruit juice. Juice does not contain the bulk or fiber of whole fruit, so it does not stabilize blood sugar or have beneficial effects on bowel function. Juice acts more like the simple sugars found in candy, so it should be used sparingly.

Seeds and Nuts

Seeds and nuts are excellent sources of protein. They are very high in calories, so quantities should be consumed in moderation. Nuts are very high in magnesium and calcium, which is important in preventing osteoporosis. They are also high in potassium, so they are highly nutritious foods. Excellent nuts for menopausal women include almonds, pecans, walnuts, and filberts; seeds include sunflower, pumpkin, and sesame seeds. Nuts and seeds should be refrigerated so their oils do not become rancid.

Unfortunately, most people eat nuts as a snack much like potato chips or taco chips. These nuts tend to be roasted and salted, both of which treatments are unhealthy. I recommend eating nuts and seeds raw and unsalted. They can be eaten as a main source of protein in a light meal, used as a garnish in salads, casseroles, and vegetable dishes.

Meat, Poultry, and Fish

The typical American meal has traditionally been centered around large portions of meat. Big steaks, chops, and oversized sandwiches are the normal serving size in most restaurants and at most family meals. While I certainly recommend retaining meat in your diet if you enjoy its flavor, the serving sizes should be dramatically reduced for women at mid-life. Most of us need only small servings (3 oz. or even less per day) to maintain an adequate protein intake. Instead of large meat portions, I recommend increasing the servings of grains, beans, and vegetables. Meat can also be used more as a garnish and flavoring for soups, casseroles and stir-fries. Meat tends to be high in saturated fat, which can increase the risk of breast and colon cancer, as well as heart disease and stroke, common diseases after mid-life. I recommend fish or poultry with the skin removed because they are leaner and have a lower fat content. Eat red meats less frequently, perhaps once a week or less, and then only in small amounts. When buying red meat, be sure to purchase lean cuts and have your butcher trim off all excess fat. Meat is hard to digest for the aging digestive tract, which is why many people feel tired after a meal with a large meat portion. Be sure to avoid completely such processed meats as ham, bologna, and salami, as they are high in fat, salt, and preservatives.

Oils

Preferred oils include flax oil, sesame oil, olive oil, corn oil, canola oil, and safflower oil. Unlike animal fats, they are unsaturated. (All except olive oil are polyunsaturated.) Cold-pressed oils tend to be fresher and purer. Wheat germ oil is are excellent source of vitamin E, as are soybean oil and corn oil.

Vitamin E has long been recognized for its effects on the female reproductive tract. It has been shown to control hot flashes and heal the vaginal and urinary tract, which can become dry, easily traumatized, and prone to infection after menopause. In fact, wheat germ oil was used for its high vitamin E content after World War II to help restore the menstrual period of women who had been interned in war camps and who had stopped menstruating due to poor nutrition and emotional shock.

Oils should be used in small quantities for cooking, sautéing, and stir-frying, except for flax oil that, because of its perishability, needs to be added to cooked food just before serving. Cold-pressed vegetable oils are also excellent in salad dressings and marinades. Refrigerate oils after opening to maintain their freshness.

Foods to Avoid

Salt

Women in the menopause years need to watch carefully their salt intake because salt can worsen high blood pressure, bloating, and fluid retention, and can contribute to osteoporosis. Unfortunately, large amounts of salt are found throughout the American diet as table salt (sodium chloride), MSG (monosodium glutamate), and a variety of food additives. Fast foods such as hamburgers, hot dogs, french fries, pizza, and tacos are loaded with salt and saturated fats. Common grocery store foods such as soups, potato chips, cheese, olives, salad dressings, and catsup (to name only a few) are also loaded with salt. And if this were not bad enough, many people use too much salt in their cooking and seasoning. Clearly, this is not healthy for anyone and can adversely affect the health of women during the menopause years.

Luckily, there are many easy and effective solutions to the salt problem. Fruits, vegetables, meat, and grains contain all the salt we need in our diet, so you can throw away your salt shaker. For flavor, use seasonings like garlic, herbs, spices, and lemon juice. Avoid processed foods that are high in salt such as canned foods, olives, pickles, potato chips, tortilla chips, catsup, salad dressings, and other high-salt foods. It is important to read labels and look for the word sodium (salt). If it appears high on the list of ingredients, don't buy the product. Many brands in the health food stores contain foods labeled "no salt added." Examples of these brands are Hain and Health Valley. Some supermarkets also contain "no added salt" foods in their diet section. Be sure to eat plenty of fresh fruits and vegetables. They are delicious, available in great variety in most supermarkets, and are full of potassium. Potassium helps to remove sodium from the body and to bring down the blood pressure.

Sugar

Most Americans eat too much sugar—the average American eats 120 pounds per year. As with salt, sugar is everywhere. Many convenience foods such as salad dressing, catsup, and relish contain high levels of both sugar and salt. Sugar is in soft drinks and in such desserts as candy, cookies, cakes, and ice cream. Many people are actually addicted to sugar and use sweet foods as a way to deal with frustration and other upsets.

The negative health effects of all this sugar show up dramatically after menopause. Excess sugar intake accelerates diabetes and blood sugar imbalances, both of which increase after menopause. Sugar depletes the body's B-complex vitamins and minerals, which can worsen nervous tension and anxiety (a real problem for some women during menopause). Highly sugared foods also promote tooth loss through tooth and gum disease.

To reduce sugar craving and excessive intake, try to satisfy your sweet tooth with healthier foods such as fruits or grain-based treats like oatmeal cookies made with fruit or honey. You will find that smaller amounts of these foods satisfy your cravings. Instead of disrupting your sugar metabolism, they actually have a healthful and balancing effect.

Caffeine

Caffeine is a stimulant found in coffee, black tea, many soft drinks, and in chocolate. Women drink caffeinated beverages to increase their energy and alertness and decrease fatigue. Unfortunately, caffeine has many negative effects on the body. Caffeine can cause breast tenderness. Fifteen to 30 percent of women with breast tenderness note relief upon eliminating caffeinated beverages. Caffeine used in excess also increases anxiety, irritability, and mood swings. This can be a real problem for some women during menopause. It also depletes the body's stores of vitamin B complex, thus interfering with carbohydrate metabolism. Many menopausal women also complain that caffeine increases the number of hot flashes. Heavy caffeine intake can also worsen osteoporosis.

With all of these negative side-effects, it is important for menopausal women to either cut down dramatically on caffeine intake or eliminate it entirely. Because cutting out caffeine can cause withdrawal symptoms such as irritability and headaches, I recommend that women eliminate caffeine gradually. To start, mix ½ cup regular coffee and ½ cup decaffeinated coffee. I recommend using water-process decaffeinated coffee, which is extracted with hot water rather than chemicals. After a month or two on decaffeinated coffee, switch to grain-based coffee substitutes such as Pero, Postum, or Caffix. Because they have a calming effect, herbal teas such as camomile and hops can actually be therapeutic for women with anxiety.

Alcohol

Alcohol should be consumed only in small amounts by menopausal women. When used carefully, not exceeding 4 oz. of wine per day, 10 oz. of beer, or 1 oz. of hard liquor, it can have a delightfully relaxing effect. It makes us more sociable and enhances the taste of food. For optimal health, however, I recommend using alcohol only as an occasional treat, not more than once or twice a week. Some women who are particularly susceptible to negative effects of alcohol shouldn't drink it at all. Alcohol depletes the body's vitamin B complex and minerals and disrupts carbohydrate metabolism. Alcohol is toxic to the liver and can disrupt the liver's ability to metabolize hormones, as well as worsen hot flashes. It has also been associated with osteoporosis in post-menopausal women. In large amounts, alcohol can be toxic to the heart and nervous system.

If you enjoy alcohol and social drinking, I recommend decreasing your total alcohol intake and exploring non-alcoholic beverages. For example, light wine and beer in small amounts have a lower alcohol content than hard liquor, liqueurs, and regular wine. A non-alcoholic cocktail such as mineral water with a twist of lime or lemon or a dash of bitters is an even better substitute. "Near beer," a non-alcoholic beer substitute, tastes like the real thing.

Dairy Products

Dairy products are high in calcium, but because of the many negative health aspects of using dairy products, I generally recommend that menopausal women avoid them and use alternative sources of calcium. Most dairy products tend to be high in saturated fat and salt content, which increase the incidence of heart attacks, strokes, and high blood pressure. Many women are allergic to dairy products or lack the enzymes to digest milk. Milk causes digestive problems in many people, including bowel changes, bloat, and gas. I have seen many women patients whose digestive problems have cleared up just by stopping milk intake. If you have menopause-related tiredness and depression, avoid cow's milk, because the tryptophan in cow's milk products increases fatigue. Finally, recent medical studies suggest that women with a high intake of dairy products suffer from a greater incidence of ovarian cancer, an often deadly disease.

I generally recommend that women use calcium, magnesium, and vitamin D supplements instead of dairy products. There are many other good sources of calcium including green leafy vegetables (collard, kale, mustard greens), beans, peas, soybeans, sesame seeds, carob, fish, and chicken stock made with bones. For food preparation, soy milk and nut milks (available at most health food stores) are good sources of calcium. They can be used for drinking, eating with cereal or baking. See the Cookbook section for high-calcium sesame and nut milks.

Fats

Americans consume 40 percent of their calories in fat. Most of these calories come from dairy products (such as butter, cream, and cheese), fatty meats (such as beef and pork), and saturated oils found in many processed foods. A high-fat diet is dangerous for menopausal women because fat is linked to heart disease, high blood pressure, stroke, and cancer of the ovaries, breast, uterus, and colon. Women on a high-fat diet also tend to accumulate more excess weight.

Instead of high-fat foods, eat more fruits, vegetables, grains, fish, and poultry. Red meat should be used less often and, when used at all, it should be lean and trimmed of fat. Cook sparingly with oil using small amounts to sauté and stir-fry foods instead of deep-frying them. Avoid complicated and rich recipes demanding large amounts of butter, cream, cheese, or other high-fat foods in the preparation. Learn to make and prepare low-fat marinades and sauces or avoid them altogether by flavoring food with garlic, onions, herbs, lemon juice, or a little olive oil (a monosaturated fat which doesn't increase your cholesterol level). Eat raw seeds and nuts rather than cooked ones (cooking alters the nature of the oils), and use them sparingly because of their high fat content. As often as possible, try to eat fresh and homemade foods made with a minimum of fats and oils. If you must eat packaged and processed foods, read the labels. Avoid those with a high fat content or added fat.

Other Basic Principles of the Menopause Self Help Diet

Eat the greatest possible variety of foods. By rotating your foods, you also minimize symptoms of food allergy. This guarantees that you will be taking in a large range of nutrients, which is very important during the menopause years and beyond to maintain optimal health. Don't fall into the rut of eating the same foods day after day. Many women will go to the same shelves of the supermarket out of habit and convenience. Eating from a small range of foods can adversely affect your health in the long run.

Keep your meals simple and easy to prepare. Women today live very busy lives. Many have the responsibility of running households and holding full-time jobs. This does not leave much time for planning and cooking meals. It is no wonder so many women turn to convenience foods. Fortunately, nutritious foods can be just as convenient as less nutritious foods. Over the years, my patients and I have worked out many shortcuts for preparing high-quality food. Many of them have used these shortcuts to great advantage, and can prepare a complete meal in ten to twenty minutes. Quick and easy-to-follow meal plans and recipes are given in the following chapters.

Healthy meals for menopause can be enjoyed with friends and family. The nutritional suggestions made in this book for optimal health during the menopause years can be used with benefit by all your family and friends. Most of my patients find that their families enjoy sharing the new foods and they feel healthier. Most dishes can be easily adapted to everyone's taste. If you still have children at home, your diet can be easily modified to fit their tastes. For example, add extra cheese and hamburger to one side of a casserole. Or prepare your side of a dish without the rich gravy that the rest of your family likes, or add more vegetables.

Eat a big breakfast and a lighter lunch and dinner. Women during the menopause years often notice a decrease in the efficiency of their digestive tract. Constipation, gas, and other intestinal upsets may be more common. Eat most of your food earlier in the day when your body is active and more efficient. Avoid eating large meals at night. Digesting food while you are asleep puts a large metabolic load on your entire system. The night is the time when your body repairs itself; it is unhealthy during this rest period to ask your body to continue to work.

Make the transition to a healthy menopause diet slowly. I have found in my medical practice that it takes anywhere from a month to two years to change one's dietary habits so that these changes feel comfortable and pleasurable (not just healthy). It is unrealistic to expect that you will throw away every high-stress food in your cupboard because of your body's changing needs.

Review the list of foods to avoid (page 43) given earlier in this chapter. Pick one or two foods from this list that you would be willing to give up immediately. Then look at the list of foods to substitute. For example, if you drink six cups of coffee a day, you might decide to switch to a coffee substitute like Postum. You may not want to make any other changes until a month later. When you are comfortable with these changes, go back to your list of foods to avoid. Perhaps now you are ready to cut down on your intake of dairy products; you could eliminate the slice of cheese from your sandwich at lunch. Instead of yogurt, you might take a bowl of soup.

Every few weeks go back to the list of foods to limit and foods to emphasize. Pick a few more foods to eliminate and a few more to add to your diet. Remember that even modest dietary changes can bring significant health improvements. On the other hand, some people find it easier to change their diets by giving up foods abruptly, and that is fine too. The important thing is to find the way that will work for you.

The Menopause Self Help Diet should be fun. The dietary suggestions in this book offer a chance to taste new types of food and try out new recipes. Approach tasting new foods as you would go to a new restaurant—with a sense of excitement and pleasure. To maximize your enjoyment of your new diet, emphasize the aesthetics of dining. A tablecloth, candles, and attractive serving dishes can dress up even simple fare. Highlight the color and texture of each food by using side dishes for serving. Try to serve foods with complementary colors. You will be widening your choice of nutrients as well as increasing the eye appeal. (For example, red and yellow vegetables are high in vitamin A, while green vegetables are higher in vitamin C.) This attention to the pleasure of dining will increase your emotional gratification and sense of well-being.

FOODS TO EAT

Fruits
Vegetables
Whole grains
Beans
Seeds and nuts
Fish
Poultry (in moderation)
Oils
Seafood (in moderation)

FOODS TO AVOID

Sugar
Salt
Fats
Caffeine
Alcohol (except in moderation)
Dairy products
Meat (except in moderation)

MENOPAUSE SHOPPING LIST

Vegetables

artichokes
avocados
beans
beets
broccoli
brussels sprouts
cabbage
carrots
celery
chard
collard greens
cucumbers
garlic
horseradish
kale
lettuce
mushrooms
mustard greens
okra
onions
parsnips
peas
potatoes
radishes
rutabagas
spinach
squash
sweet potatoes
tomatoes
turnip greens
turnips
yams

Whole Grains

barley
brown rice
buckwheat
corn
millet
oatmeal
rye
wild rice

Seeds and Nuts

almonds
filberts
flax
peanuts
pecans
pumpkin seeds
sesame seeds
sunflower seeds

Fruits

apples
apricots
bananas
berries
grapefruit
kiwi fruits
lemons
melons
oranges
papayas
peaches
pears
pineapples
plums

Oils

canola
corn
flax
olive
sesame
safflower
sunflower

Meats

fish
poultry (in moderation)
seafood (in moderation)

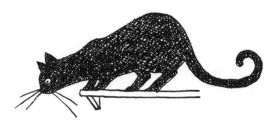

CHAPTER 6

Menus and Meal Plans

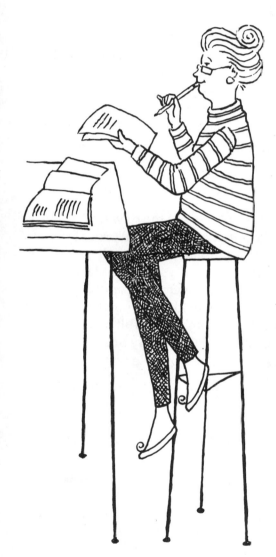

I have found over the years that most of my patients want specific guidelines on menus and meal plans. Although it is tremendously helpful to provide information on the foods to eat and foods to avoid, most women want to know how to make the next step and combine the right foods in healthful meals. They also want to know how to make the transition from their old diet to a new program without too much difficulty or confusion. I found that thousands of my patients benefited enormously from these simple and easy-to-follow guidelines, so I have included the information in this chapter for your benefit, too.

General Guidelines

Make All Dietary Changes Gradually

The transition to a healthful menopause diet should be done in an easy and non-stressful manner. Don't try to change all of your dietary habits at once by making a clean sweep of your refrigerator and pantry. I've seen patients do that and come to my office in an absolute panic.

I recommend instead that you substitute several healthy foods for high-stress foods that you have been eating. To do this, periodically review the lists of foods to limit and foods to emphasize. Each time you review this list, pick several foods that you are willing to eliminate and several to try. Review these lists as often as you choose, but try to do it on a regular basis. Every small change that you make in your diet can help.

Keep Your Meals Simple and Easy to Prepare

Many women lead busy, active lives and don't have a lot of time to cook complicated meals. For that reason, I've kept my meal plans quick and simple to prepare, with the main emphasis on foods that are delicious and high in nutrition. For those who are used to eating quick meals at fast-food restaurants or commercial snack food that is high in fat, sugar, and food additives, these simple meals offer a much healthier alternative.

Breakfast

Breakfast is actually the most important meal of the day. If you choose foods that are healthful and nourishing, they will provide the energy you need for the vigor and vitality to sail through your work and activities. Unfortunately, many women skip breakfast entirely. Others eat foods like doughnuts and coffee in hopes of getting quick energy, but these foods can instead make you tense and anxious. Other women may eat hearty breakfasts full of high-stress foods—eggs, bacon, milk, toast, and butter. Any one of these meals can wreak havoc for women in menopause years. The breakfast plan should include:

Beverages

Adequate liquid intake is very important. Use beverages that provide important nutrients and make you feel calm and relaxed throughout the day. These include fruit juices, herbal teas, roasted grain beverages (coffee substitutes), nondairy milks, and spring water. Fruit juices make an excellent breakfast drink because of their high levels of vitamin C, vitamin A, potassium, and other essential nutrients. Good herbal teas for breakfast include camomile and hops, which can calm your nerves if you tend to be anxious or edgy in the morning. Ginger is an excellent choice for women who tend to be tired in the morning and need a pick-me-up. Other healthful teas include blackberry, raspberry, and peppermint. Grain-based coffee substitutes, such as Postum, Pero, or Caffix, are hearty, satisfying beverages.

I strongly recommmend that coffee drinkers switch to these beverages to avoid the stressful effects of caffeine. The same pick-me-up can be accomplished in a much better way through the use of proper herbs, vitamins and minerals, and exercise. Decaffeinated coffee in small amounts may be used as a transition beverage while making the switch to herbal teas or coffee substitutes. Nondairy milk like soy, nut, or grain milk can be delicious, both as an occasional beverage or in cereal. Soy milk is now easy to find in health food stores. Nut milks can be made easily and quickly in a blender and are delicious (see Recipe section). The most important drink of all is water, 6 to 8 glasses per day. I recommend that you use spring or filtered tap water. With the increasing pollution of our groundwater, water purity is becoming a real health concern. Until this trend is reversed through adequate protection of our water supply, I recommend staying away from drinking tap water if at all possible, or buying a filter for home use.

Fruits

Fruits make a wonderful breakfast food because they are great sources of such vitamins and minerals as vitamin C, vitamin A, and potassium. While fruits are high in sugar content, they are also high in fiber. This makes us feel full faster and decreases our appetite so we don't overeat. The fiber in fruit also helps to regulate bowel function, an important plus for women in menopause who commonly complain of sluggish bowel function. For most women, a wide variety of fruits are available year-round, particularly apples, bananas, oranges, and grapefruit. These staples of the American diet are great breakfast foods. It is also a good idea to enjoy the seasonal fruits such as apricots, peaches, berries, cherries, melons, and the other delicious fruits available only for a short time during the year. Try to eat locally grown fruits in season, as they will tend to be riper and fresher. Also, try to find unsprayed and organic fruit, if possible, to avoid pesticide exposure. Many supermarkets are beginning to carry unsprayed foods because of the strong consumer demand for clean products.

Whole Grain Foods

These are among your best breakfast foods. Whole grain foods are high in vitamin B complex, magnesium, potassium, and vitamin E. They are high in complex carbohydrates, which are the best foods to stabilize your blood sugar and provide constant, slowly released energy throughout the day. Complex carbohydrates also help tremendously to normalize the mood swings and anxiety that some women suffer from during menopause. These foods include:

Hot Cereals. As I mentioned in the last chapter, rice, rye, and oats are other grains I prefer over wheat cereals because of wheat's tendency to cause allergies, bloating, and digestive upset. Your local health food store will have a wide range of excellent grain cereals available. Look for cream of rye, cream of buckwheat, whole grain oatmeal, and seven- or four-grain cereals (without wheat). Choose brands without added sugar. If there is no health food store near you, most supermarkets will have adequate products. I highly recomend Quaker whole oatmeal (not the quick-cooking refined product). Many of the "natural cereals" from the large companies are either highly refined or highly sugared, so read the labels carefully and watch out. Many supermarkets are beginning to carry bulk cereals in bins. Perhaps a grocery store near you has these products available.

Cold Cereals. Again, there are a large number available in the health food stores, including puffed rice, corn, or millet, and unsweetened granola. At supermarkets look for products that say "whole grain." Avoid cold cereals with added sugar.

You can moisten your cereal with a very small amount of cow's milk or use substitutes such as goat's milk, soy milk, or nut milk.

Some women enjoy eating cold cereals dry or with a small amount of apple juice. For sweeteners your best bet is fructose or maple syrup. They are very concentrated in flavor, so a little bit goes a long way.

Muffins, Breads, and Crackers. It is easy to find in the supermarkets or to prepare delicious whole grain breads, muffins, and crackers. I have included several examples in the Cookbook section. I recommend oat muffins with extra oat bran, rye muffins, or corn bread. Also highly recommended are the rice cakes commonly available at health food stores and now increasingly stocked at neighborhood supermarkets. Wheat-free bread can be found in the health food stores. Muffins, bread, and crackers can be eaten with applesauce, nut butter, fruit, preserves, or a small amount of margarine. Try to avoid cow's milk butter, which is high in saturated fat.

Spreads. Peanut butter (without added salt), sesame butter (which is high in calcium), and soy spreads are good spreads. Sesame butter is in the foreign foods department of most supermarkets and is available in all health food stores. It is delicious and a wonderful source of nutrients. It is also very filling, so a little bit goes a long way. Applesauce and fruit preserves made without sugar are also good on toast, pancakes, and muffins.

Breakfast Menus

These easy-to-prepare menus will provide a variety of healthful and delicious meals. They can also act as guidelines for you to create your own meal plans. Recipes for many of these foods (see asterisk) can be found in the Cookbook section.

Oatmeal with maple syrup*	Brown rice waffles*
Apple	Blackberries
Peppermint tea*	Roasted grain beverage (coffee substitute)
Muesli*	
Sunflower seeds	Fruit smoothie*
Orange-strawberry juice*	Almonds and raisins
Corn bread*	Whole grain bread
Pear	Tofu/peanut butter spread
Hot carob drink*	Piña colada juice*
Rye muffins*	Puffed rice cereal
Apple-spice butter	Soy milk
Sesame milk*	Banana

Lunch and Dinner

Soups

Soups are an excellent food because they can combine a variety of such highly nutritious ingredients as vegetables, grains, starches, meat, and fish. Soups can also be easy to prepare because the ingredients can be combined and then cooked relatively unattended while you do other things. I highly recommend homemade soups, since you can avoid salt, high fat content, and food additives in the preparation. I have included a number of simple and delicious soup recipes in the Cookbook section. If you buy canned or powdered soup, use the "no added salt or sugar" types. Hain and Health Valley brands make soups labeled "no added salt," which are easy to find in the health food stores. If there is no health food store near you, read the soup product labels in your supermarket carefully.

I strongly recommend legume soups such as lentil or split pea with a grain product (cereal, toast). This combination provides excellent sources of protein: grains and legumes complement each other in their amino acid content and together produce a high-quality protein. Also good are vegetable soup and chicken broth. If you are concerned about osteoporosis, add chicken, fish, or veal bones to your soup base along with a few tablespoons of vinegar. The vinegar will pull calcium from the bones and give you a nice rich soup. For women who can't eat soup without some salt flavor, I would suggest adding one teaspoon of miso to your cup of soup. Miso is a fermented soy product of Japanese origin. It is easily found in Oriental markets and health food stores. It is much lower in salt content than regular table salt.

Salads

Salads are a wonderful source of light eating and varied nutrition. Many vegetables contain the nutrients essential for women during the menopause years. For example, many greens are high in magnesium, calcium, and iron, while beans are high in calcium. The more adventuresome you are in your salad making, the more likely you are to have a highly nutritious meal. For example, don't stick to iceberg lettuce as your salad base. Dark green vegetables such as fresh spinach, romaine lettuce, endive, parsley, and red lettuce are more nutritious than iceberg lettuce and make a beautiful presentation. Salads can be made from a variety of raw vegetables. Use turnips, beets, green beans, radishes, carrots, cauliflower, avocados, red peppers, water chestnuts, zucchini, snow peas, and jicama. They can be garnished with sprouts, soy bits, seeds, croutons, and nuts. Cooked beans such as kidney, pinto, and garbanzo are great sources of protein when added to your salad. A small amount of shrimp or fish can be added for a more filling salad. Avoid store-bought salad dressings. Many contain MSG, sugar, and undesirable chemicals and oils. Your own can be made with cold-pressed oils, lemon juice, or vinegar. Add the dressing just before serving or serve it on the side so that the diners can choose their own. Avoid the thick, creamy dressings that are high in calories and fat.

Sandwiches

For many busy women, a well-put-together sandwich is a quick, easy, and delicious meal. The filling should contain a variety of nutritious vegetables such as lettuce, tomatoes, onion, sprouts, and avocados used either as garnishes or as the sandwich base. Lean meat such as turkey, chicken (without the skin), and water-pack tuna are high in protein and low in calories. Also good are bean spreads such as soy, hummus, and tahini (made from garbanzo beans and sesame seeds). Avoid rich, buttery breads for your sandwiches such as croissants and brioches. For example, the average croissant is over 50 percent butterfat. Also avoid high-fat fillings such as cheese, cream cheese, sausage, hot dogs, bologna and salami, or rich dressings, such as Thousand Island dressings. These are difficult to digest, dangerous for your cardiovascular system, and can cause excess weight gain.

Vegetables

These should be eaten raw or lightly steamed for optimal nutrition. They are an important accompaniment to main courses like grains, beans, meat, and fish, and can help to balance your meals properly. Don't boil, cook in heavy oil, or cover vegetables with sauce. The high nutrient value of the vegetables is either lost or compromised with high-stress ingredients. Excellent vegetables for women in the menopause years include:

Leafy green vegetables. Kale, spinach, collard, turnip greens, mustard greens, and beet greens are packed with nutrients such as calcium, magnesium, and iron. Greens should be lightly steamed (never boiled) until tender but not soggy. After steaming, dress them with a mixture of olive oil, lemon juice and a touch of sea salt.

Broccoli, brussels sprouts, and cauliflower. They are delicious steamed and lightly dressed with lemon juice. Broccoli can also be eaten raw or used in salads.

Root vegetables. Rutabagas, turnips, parsnips, beets, and sweet potatoes are packed with important vitamins and minerals. They can be steamed or baked and served whole, mashed or julienned (cut into long strips like french fries). Many women eat these vegetables rarely or only on holidays. I would recommend enjoying them much more often.

Squash. This delicious vegetable is easy to digest and is low in calories. Baking squash makes it dry and stringy. There are two better ways to prepare it:

- Steam until soft, then puree the squash in a blender. The resulting puree will be soft, smooth, and a beautiful golden color. The pureeing breaks down the complex carbohydrates so that it is surprisingly sweet and delicious—the taste is similar to sweet potatoes. You may want to add nutmeg and cinnamon for flavor.
- Slice the squash and sauté in olive oil, soy sauce, or broth.

Carrots and celery. These are members of the same food family. Both are delicious eaten raw, especially if kept crisp and chilled. They are also tasty when sliced and steamed. Eat carrots with a small amount of maple syrup to enhance their own sweetness. Celery is delicious with onions or parsley.

Cabbage. This vegetable is delicious when chopped into a slaw or steamed. For an elegant but simple presentation, cut the cabbage in half, then cut wedges out of the cabbage like slices of a pie. Steam these wedges and serve each wedge on its own small side plate. Sprinkle with parsley, fennel, or caraway seeds.

Grains, Starches, and Legumes

Served together, these foods can be used as the chief source of complex carbohydrates and proteins for your lunch or dinner.

Grains and beans are filling, slow to digest, and tend to stabilize the blood sugar level. They are excellent foods for women with diabetes (an increasingly common problem after menopause) or blood sugar imbalances. Many women are discouraged from cooking beans and grains because of the preparation time. Here is a method to speed up the cooking time for beans:

Bring water to a boil (three cups of water for every cup of beans). Add the beans to the boiling water and cook for two minutes. Remove from the heat, partially cover the pan, and let beans stand for one hour. Go about your business or chores during this time as the beans are cooking themselves. After one hour, drain and rinse with cold water and then freeze. When you are ready to use the beans for a meal, thaw them quickly under running water. Boil five cups of water in a pot for every cup of beans. Add the beans. Lower the heat and then cook for thirty to fifty minutes. The beans will then be ready to use.

Brown rice or grains. These can be prepared in large quantities. Grains store for several days in the refrigerator in a jar or plastic container. They can be reheated and used as needed for dishes. Rice is best reheated by placing it over a double boiler or in a steamer and cooking it for three to five minutes.

Potatoes. Potatoes are extremely easy to digest if baked or steamed. The problem with potatoes is the garnishes many people use, such as butter, sour cream, and bacon. These high-fat garnishes should be avoided; use chives, sunflower seeds, and other no-salt seasonings instead. Potatoes can also be stuffed with leftover vegetables with broth added for extra flavor.

Meat and Fish

Serve steamed or roasted (without skin for poultry). Avoid heavy sauces or dressings. Always get lean cuts and trim off all visible fat. Fish and poultry should be eaten more frequently than beef, pork, or lamb, which are higher in fat content. American dinners traditionally have been organized around a large piece of meat or fish, which formed the focal point, with small servings of grain and vegetables as side dishes. For women who want to enjoy optimal health during the menopause years, I recommend reversing the ratio. Keep your meat portions small (3 oz) and fill up with a variety of other nutritious side dishes. Most people eat much more meat protein than necessary. In large quantities, meat is hard to digest and can increase fatigue in many women.

Combination Plates

In these dishes, a variety of foods are combined for both ease of preparation and taste. Vegetables and grains are the main ingredients, with meat used more as a flavoring (cut into small pieces and added to soups, salads, casseroles, and stir-fried dishes). Examples of combination plates would include chicken soup with rice and vegetables, or tacos with beans, shredded chicken, or shrimp on a corn tortilla. With added vegetables and sauce, the taco provides three good sources of high-quality protein: meat, beans, and grain. Casseroles should not be made with cheese or butter-based sauces, but with more nutritious sauces. For example, puree vegetables such as broccoli, cauliflower, or carrots, and then blend the puree with chicken broth for a creamy sauce. Arrowroot powder, rice flour, or buckwheat flakes can be added as a thickener. Tofu can also be blended into the sauce for extra creaminess.

Spices

Avoid black pepper, table salt, sugar, and monosodium glutamate (MSG), which are highly stressful to the body. Instead, use the milder herbs such as basil, thyme, dill, and tarragon. If you must use the stronger spices, use only one-half to one-fourth the amount called for in the recipe.

Lunch and Dinner Menus

These menus give you a variety of ways to organize your meals. Use them as guidelines to make your own menus. The recipes for many of these dishes (indicated by asterisk) are provided in the Cookbook section.

SOUP MEALS

Split-pea soup*
Corn bread*
Green salad*
Apple sauce*

Potassium broth*
Rye bread
Sliced tomatoes
Melon slices

Tomato soup*
Steamed potato
Green beans
Pear

Lentil soup*
Wild rice
Broccoli with lemon
Romaine salad*
Pound cake

SANDWICH MEALS

Tuna salad sandwich*
Rye bread
Cole slaw

Vegetarian sandwich
Rice bread
Potato salad*
Apple

Almond butter and jam*
Whole grain bread
Vegetable broth*
Sliced bananas

Avocado sandwich*
Pita bread
Celery and carrot sticks
Oatmeal cookies

SALAD MEALS

Calcium salad*
French dressing
Lentil soup*
Whole grain bread

Apple and walnut salad
Celery sticks
Rye muffins*

Guacamole with fresh
    vegetables*
Corn chips
Fresh fruit combo

Carrot-raisin salad*
Potato salad*
Green bean salad*
Tea cookies

MEAT MEALS

Broiled trout with dill*
Steamed Italian green beans
Baked potato
Mixed green salad*

Grilled sole
Broccoli and turnips
Watercress salad*

Poached halibut*
Brown rice*
Peas and carrots*
Cole slaw

Roast turkey
Corn soya bread*
Carrots and onions*
Cauliflower and parsley*
Acorn squash dessert*

Grilled tuna
Wild rice
Steamed asparagus

Poached salmon*
Steamed artichoke*
Broccoli with lemon

ONE-DISH MEALS

Tofu with snow peas*
Melon slices

Tacos*
Guacamole with fresh
  vegetables*
Tomato and avocado garnish

Tofu and brown rice*
Zucchini with scallions and
  garlic

Chop suey*
Brown rice*
Papaya and pineapple

Healthy Breakfast Options

- Beverages
- Fruit
- Grains—cereals, muffins, and bread
- Spreads
- Raw nuts and seeds

Healthy Lunch and Dinner Options

- Beverages—mineral water, light wine or beer, herbal tea, juice, roasted grain beverage
- Soup
- Salad and dressing
- Sandwich
- Grains and starches
- Vegetables
- Fish, poultry
- One-dish meals
- Low-stress dessert

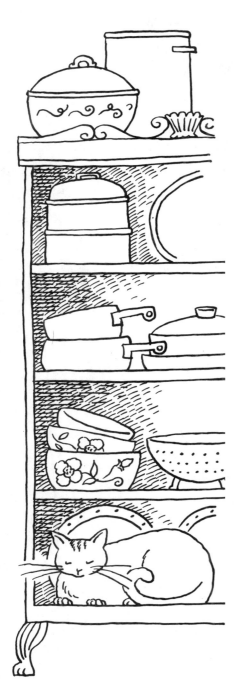

CHAPTER 7

The Healthy Kitchen

Cooking for menopause should be easy and quick, as well as beneficial for your health. I don't believe that cooking should be a complicated affair with endless preparation and all sorts of special and expensive kitchen equipment. In this chapter I will describe the few pieces of equipment that I think will make your life in the kitchen easier. I will also discuss the best cooking techniques to use and how to substitute ingredients in recipes. This information has paid off in health benefits for me and my patients over the years.

Cooking Equipment

There are several pieces of equipment that can make your food preparation simple and easy:

Stainless Steel Steamer. Steaming is highly recommended as a way to cook vegetables, fruits, and meat. No extra fat is used in the cooking process. The vitamin and mineral content of your food is retained in the cooking process; this is not the case in boiling, where essential nutrients are leached from the food.

Wok. A wok can be used to fry food with a minimum of oil. In fact, usually the fat in the meat or vegetables is all that is needed, along with a little water or broth for cooking. Delicious one-dish meals using meat, grains, and vegetables can be made in a few minutes.

Blender. A blender can be used to make nondairy milk, smoothies, sauces, and purees of fruits and vegetables. A blender is relatively inexpensive and is a quick and easy way to prepare many high-nutrient foods.

Food Processor. Salads, slaws, dough, and other foods requiring chopping, grating, and shredding can be made rapidly with a food processor.

Stainless Steel, Glass, Enamel, or Iron Pots and Pans. Avoid using aluminum or copper cookware, as the metal can leach into your food. Acid foods interact with aluminum to form aluminum salts, which are toxic. Aluminum has been implicated in Alzheimer's disease, a disorder of the nervous system that impairs intellectual faculties and memory. When buying enamel cookware be careful to buy a high quality brand, as inferior enamel can chip away and expose the underlying metal. Cooking with iron, however, may actually provide useful supplemental iron for menopausal women who have lost iron over a lifetime of menstruating.

Healthy Food Preparation and Cooking Techniques

All women in the menopause years should be knowledgeable about healthy methods of food preparation and beneficial cooking techniques. Proper food preparation that decreases the amount of high-stress ingredients in your meals can decrease your risk of cancer and heart disease. Healthy cooking techniques can also make the difference between extra fats, calories, and many unwanted pounds. How you cook and prepare food is just as important for good health and disease prevention as using fresh and wholesome ingredients.

How to Prepare Fruits and Vegetables

Fruits and vegetables should be clean and fresh. Try to avoid produce that has been sprayed with dangerous pesticides. There have been many stories in the news lately about people becoming sick on heavily sprayed food. These chemicals accumulate in our bodies and weaken our immune systems. Many health food stores now carry unsprayed produce and, increasingly, so do the large grocery store chains. Call stores in your area and look for advertisements in your local newspapers for clean foods. If none is available locally, I recommend washing produce thoroughly in water and liquid soap to at least wash off the surface residues of pesticides.

Buy fruits and vegetables in season. These tend to be products grown locally. They will be fresher, more tender, and more flavorful than produce grown out of season and shipped from far away.

Store fresh produce carefully in the crisper drawer of your refrigerator to keep fresh. Potatoes, onion, and garlic should be stored in cool dark areas to stay fresh. Shop more frequently so that your produce is fresher.

Fresh produce is the best for optimal nutrition. Canned and frozen produce loses essential nutrients in preparation and does compare in flavor or quality.

Fresh fruits and vegetables can be served whole or, for attractive presentation, can be diced, julienned, or chopped and served fresh. Carrots, celery, jicama, broccoli, cauliflower, cabbage, spinach, tomato, cucumber, mushroom, and many other vegetables are delicious when served raw. They look lovely on the plate and are full of vitamin A, C, magnesium, calcium, and many other essential menopause nutrients. They can also be eaten with light dips or dressings. (See Cookbook section for recipes.)

To cook produce, steaming is the most effective way to guard nutrients and preserve flavor. Food to be steamed is placed in a basket above boiling water. The food is cooked by steam and doesn't touch the boiling water directly. After the water has boiled a few seconds, turn the flame low and place a lid on the pot to hold the steam in. Steamed food tends to have a much more interesting texture and taste than boiled food. Steaming takes no longer than preparing frozen vegetables or heating a TV dinner. Heavily boiled, baked, or sautéed produce is the most devoid of nutrients. These cooking techniques should be avoided.

Another effective way to cook vegetables is oil-less stir-frying. This method can replace frying in many dishes and thus eliminate a lot of fat. It can be done either in a frying pan or in a wok. Instead of hot oil, use broth, bouillon, soy sauce, or water. Stir the foods into the hot liquid. This will cook them quickly and seal the juices into the food. Many vegetables contain enough natural sugar to brown naturally by this method.

To prepare salads, ingredients should be crisp and fresh. They should be well drained in a colander or on a paper towel. Rather than cutting leaf lettuce, gently tear the leaves by hand and toss them into the salad bowl. Add the dressing just before serving or serve it on the side so that each diner can choose her own. Dark green vegetables such as romaine lettuce, endive, parsley, watercress, and red lettuce are more nutritious than iceberg lettuce. Salads can be made from a variety of raw vegetables such as turnips, beets, carrots, cauliflower, water chestnuts, snow peas, and jicama. Many of these vegetables contain high amounts of calcium and other important menopause nutrients. Cooked beans such as garbanzos (chick peas) and kidney beans are also excellent salad ingredients and provide a fine source of protein.

Store leftover salad ingredients in a well-sealed plastic bag. This insures that the vegetables remain fresh and crisp.

How to Prepare Meat, Poultry, and Seafood

Buy range-fed meat and poultry if at all possible. Many meat and poultry producers keep the animals in close, cramped quarters.

These animals are given hormones, antibiotics, and other chemicals to grow and fatten quickly. The meat is often treated chemically from the slaughterhouse to the supermarket so that the meat has a longer shelf life.

In contrast, range-fed meat and poultry is allowed to roam, eat a healthful and varied diet and to mature longer. I don't want dangerous chemical residues from meat in my body and neither should you. I have also found range-fed meat to be more tender and flavorful. Range-fed meat and poultry is available at most health food stores and increasingly in supermarket chains.

Buy lean cuts of meat. Avoid prime meat, which is more expensive and marbled with fat, or fatty cuts like chuck steak. If you eat beef, use the leaner cuts of meat like flank steak and lean hamburger. Be sure to ask the butcher to trim all the extra fat off the meat, or do this yourself at home. Poultry should have all the skin removed. This decreases significantly the calories as well as the meat's fat content.

Try to eat fish at least once or twice a week. Fish has a low fat content and contains many essential nutrients like iodine, which is essential for a healthy thyroid. It is low in calories and for many people fish is easier to digest than beef, pork, or lamb.

Avoid deep-frying or pan-frying. These methods increase the fat content of meat. If you want to fry your meat, try oil-less stir-frying. You can stir-fry meat in a frying pan or wok. Instead of cooking with hot oil, use hot water, broth, bouillon, or soy sauce. The natural fat in the meat will give a delicious taste to the meat when cooked this way.

Try cooking meat, poultry, and fish by steaming, stewing, and simmering. This way the meat can be cooked with water or vegetable juices rather than fat. Meat is tender and delicious when cooked this way and the essential nutrients are preserved.

When roasting meat such as beef roast or poultry, place the meat on a rack, spit, or stand. This enables the fat to run off. The meat should not sit in a pool of fat. This cooking technique helps to reduce the amount of saturated fat that you will be eating.

When cooking meat in the oven, bake at low to moderate temperatures (325 to 375 degrees). Slow cooking allows meat to stay moist and tender and preserves more nutrients.

Avoid heavy, thick sauces and gravies. These are full of oil, butter, cheese, and other high-stress ingredients. Serve the meat simply with a non-salt seasoning mix, herbs, or no flavor enhancers at all. This will allow you to enjoy the delicious taste of the food itself.

How to Substitute in Recipes

Cooking a healthful diet for menopause does not mean that you have to give up your favorite cookbooks and recipes. While most cookbooks use many high-stress ingredients such as dairy products and sugar to give recipes extra flavor, you can still make your favorite dishes by substituting ingredients. This will allow you to decrease the large amounts of chocolate, milk products, sugar, salt, and other foods that many recipes call for. These high-stress foods are not necessary to make food taste good, and they can even worsen menopause symptoms. You can also reduce the amount of the ingredients by a substantial amount and still retain all the flavor and taste. Most of us have palates jaded by too much salt, sugar, and other flavorings. In many dishes all we taste are the additives and never really enjoy the delicious flavor of the foods themselves. For years I have cooked by substituting ingredients; I enjoy the subtle taste of the dishes much more, and I find that my health and vitality continue to improve with the deletion of high-stress ingredients in my food. Use the following information on how to substitute healthy ingredients in your own recipes. The substitutions are easy and simple to make, and should benefit your health greatly.

How to Substitute for Sugar

Cut the amount of sweetener in your recipes by one-third to one-half. Americans tend to be addicted to sugar. That is simply a fact based on our tendency to consume close to 100 pounds of sugar a year. Most of us grew up on highly sugared soft drinks, candy, and rich pastries—no wonder the incidence of diabetes is soaring among our population. I have found that, as women decrease their sugar intake, most of them begin to really enjoy the subtle flavors of the foods they eat.

Substitute more concentrated sweeteners. Concentrated sweeteners such as honey and maple syrup have a sweeter taste per quantity used than table sugar. This will allow you to cut down on the actual amount of sugar used in a recipe. If you use a concentrated sweetener in place of sugar in an ordinary recipe, reduce the liquid content in the recipe by ¼ cup. If no liquid is used in the recipe, add 3 to 4 tablespoons of flour for each ¾ cup of concentrated sweetener.

Substitute fruit for sugar in pastries. In making muffins and cookies, you may want to try deleting sugar altogether and adding extra fruits and nuts.

How to Substitute for Dairy Products

Decrease the amount of cheese you use in cooking. If you must use cheese in cooking, decrease the amount by ½ to ⅔ so that it becomes a flavoring or garnish rather than a major source of fat and protein. Tofu can be added to the recipes to replace cheese. Try to use the lower-fat cheese now available if you cannot give up cow's milk products. However, goat's or sheep's cheese can be used to replace cow's cheese, since the fat they contain is more easily emulsified in the body.

Milk can often be easily replaced in recipes. Try substituting soy milk, nut milks, or grain milks. Soy milk and nut milks are available at most health food stores. They are good sources of calcium and can be used for drinking, eating with cereal, or baking. Add calcium to the drinks for extra menopause nutrition. (See the Cookbook section for several easy ways to make milk substitutes.) Vegetable cooking water, rice water, or potato water can be substituted for milk or cream as a thickener for sauces. (Add one cup of cooked rice or a cooked, diced potato to half a cup of water and blend in blender.)

Substitute vegetable oil spreads for butter. For women needing to watch their saturated fat intake, there are many vegetable oil products available that may be substituted for butter. Some of these products are quite tasty and have a pleasing texture. They should, however, be used only in small amounts.

How to Substitute for Salt

Substitute potassium-based products for table salt (sodium chloride). Potassium-based products are much healthier and will not aggravate heart disease or hypertension.

Substitute powdered seaweeds like kelp or nori to season vegetables, grains, and salads. They are high in essential iodine and trace elements.

Use herbs instead of salt for flavoring. Their flavor is much more subtle and will help even the most jaded palate appreciate the taste of fresh fruits, vegetables, and meats.

How to Substitute for Chocolate and Cocoa

Substitute carob for chocolate. Unsweetened carob tastes like chocolate but is far more nutritious. It is a member of the legume family and is high in calcium. It can be purchased in chunk form as a substitute for chocolate candy or as a powder to be used in baking or drinks. Be careful, however, not to overindulge: carob, like chocolate, is high in calories and fat. It should be considered a treat and an excellent cooking aid to be used only in small amounts.

How to Substitute for Coffee

Use coffee substitutes. The best substitutes for cooking are the grain-based coffee substitutes like Pero, Postum, and Caffix.

Use decaffeinated coffee as a transition beverage. For women who cannot give up coffee, start by substituting water-process decaffeinated coffee for the real thing. Then try to wean yourself from coffee altogether, or go to a coffee substitute.

How to Substitute for White Flour

Use whole grain flour. Substitute whole grain flour, which is much higher in essential nutrients like vitamin B complex and many minerals. It is also higher in fiber content.

How to Substitute for Alcohol

Use low-alcohol or non-alcoholic products for cooking. Substitute low-alcohol or non-alcoholic wine or beer when cooking or preparing sauces and marinades. You will retain much of the flavor that alcohol imparts and you'll decrease the stress factor substantially.

Substitutes for Common High-Stress Ingredients

¾ cup sugar	½ cup honey
	¼ cup molasses
	½ cup maple syrup
	½ ounces barley malt
	1 cup apple butter
	2 cups apple juice
1 cup milk	1 cup soy milk, nut milk, or grain milk. (See Cookbook section for recipes.) To make this a high-calcium drink, add 1,000 mg liquid or powdered calcium supplement and 400 I.U. vitamin D to one quart nondairy milk.

½ teaspoon salt	1 tablespoon miso
	½ teaspoon potassium chloride salt substitute
	½ teaspoon Ms. Dash, Health Valley or other non-sodium seasoning
	½ teaspoon herbs (basil, tarragon, oregano, etc.)
	½ teaspoon Bragg's liquid amino acids
	½ teaspoon sea vegetables—dulse, kelp
1½ cups cocoa	1 cup powdered carob
1 square chocolate	¾ tablespoon powdered carob
1 tablespoon coffee	1 tablespoon decaffeinated coffee
	1 tablespoon Pero, Postum, Caffix, or other grain-based coffee substitute
4 ounces wine	4 ounces light wine
8 ounces beer	8 ounces near beer
1 cup white flour	1 cup rice flour (bread, muffins, cookies)
	1 cup barley flour (pie crust)

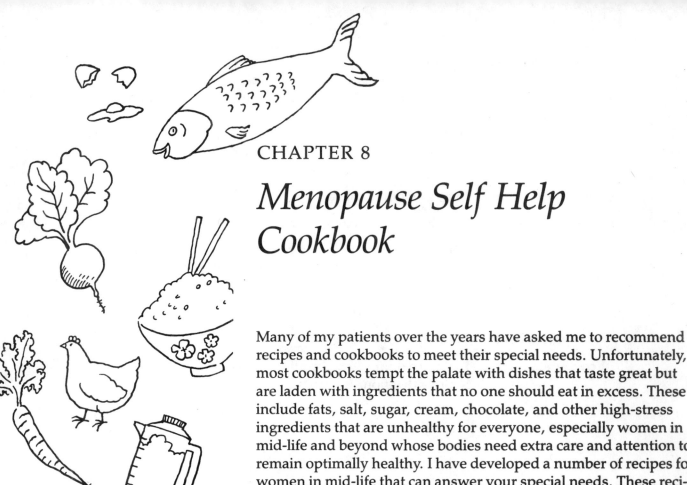

CHAPTER 8

Menopause Self Help Cookbook

Many of my patients over the years have asked me to recommend recipes and cookbooks to meet their special needs. Unfortunately, most cookbooks tempt the palate with dishes that taste great but are laden with ingredients that no one should eat in excess. These include fats, salt, sugar, cream, chocolate, and other high-stress ingredients that are unhealthy for everyone, especially women in mid-life and beyond whose bodies need extra care and attention to remain optimally healthy. I have developed a number of recipes for women in mid-life that can answer your special needs. These recipes are low in salt, fat, and sugar, and they are high in calcium, potassium, vitamin C, vitamin A, and other essential nutrients needed to rebuild and repair the body and maintain vibrant health. I have specifically included beverages, soups, salads, and desserts that are very high in calcium, since few women get enough in their normal diet. Sufficient calcium is essential to prevent osteoporosis. These recipes are simple, quick, and easy to prepare. I have found that anything too complicated doesn't work for my life and certainly won't for most of my patients. Best of all, these recipes are delicious and satisfying as well as nutritious. I hope that you will enjoy them as much as I do.

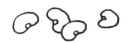

Breakfast

BEVERAGES

Fruit Smoothie
Makes 2–3 cups

1 cup orange or apple juice
2 bananas
¾ cup fresh fruit (pineapple, blackberries, blueberries, raspberries, papaya, peaches, or strawberries)

Combine apple or orange juice in a blender with bananas and your choice of a third fruit. Blend until smooth and serve.

Herb Tea
Makes 2 cups

1 teaspoon of herb leaves (fennel, peppermint, camomile, ginger, raspberry leaf, rose hips, strawberry leaf, or oat straw)
1 pint water
1 teaspoon honey (if desired)

Bring water to a boil. Place herb leaves in water. Simmer for fifteen minutes and serve.

Hot Carob Drink
Makes 1 cup

1 cup hot water
2 tablespoons carob syrup

Fill cup with hot water. Add two tablespoons carob syrup (see recipe below). This drink may be used to replace hot chocolate.

Carob Syrup
Makes 2 cups

¼ cup carob powder
1 cup water
1 cup honey
½ teaspoon vanilla
pinch salt

Combine water, honey, and carob powder in a cooking pot and bing to a rolling boil. Let cool. Add vanilla and salt. This may be stored in the refrigerator.

Sesame Milk #1

Makes 1½ cups

½ cup apple juice
½ cup water
3 ice cubes
3 tablespoons tahini (sesame butter)
½ banana
500 mg liquid or powdered calcium (if desired)

Combine all ingredients in a blender. This makes a delicious beverage.

Sesame Milk #2

Makes 2 cups

¾ cup apple juice
4 ice cubes
2 tablespoons tahini (sesame butter)
½ frozen banana
2 pitted dates
500 mg liquid or powdered calcium (if desired)

Combine all ingredients in a blender for a wonderful treat.

Almond Milk

Makes 1¼ cups

½ cup raw or blanched almonds
1 tablespoon honey or rice syrup
1 cup warm water
250 mg liquid or powdered calcium (if desired)

Combine nuts, honey, and ½ cup of warm water in a blender. Slowly add remaining water and blend until creamy. If you like a thinner milk, add 1 to 3 ounces more warm water.

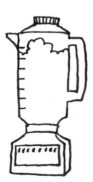

Oat Milk

Makes approximately 2 cups

¼ cup rolled oats
2 cups water
⅓ banana
¼ teaspoon cinnamon
2 ounces apple juice
pinch of salt
250 mg of liquid or powdered
   calcium (if desired)

Combine oats and hot water in a pot. Simmer in covered pot for 20 minutes. Whip in blender with remaining ingredients until smooth and creamy.

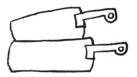

WHOLE GRAIN FOODS

Whole Grain Cereals

Serves 2

2 cups cold water
1 cup cereal (choose one or more
   grains from below)
barley   oats
buckwheat   corn
rye   rice

Put 1 cup of cereal and 2 cups of cold water in a pot. Add a pinch of salt. Heat and stir cereal constantly until it boils. Cover and turn off heat. Let stand for 20 minutes and serve.

Muesli

Serves 4

⅔ cups rolled oats
½ teaspoon ground cinnamon
⅔ cup water
½ apple, with skin
1 banana, sliced
1 cup soy or nut milk
6 chopped almonds
¼ cup raisins

Combine oats and raisins, cover with water and soak overnight. In the morning, add nuts, cinnamon, bananas, and apples to the oats. Add nut or soy milk and serve.

Rice and Oatmeal Pancakes

Serves 4 to 6

1 cup rolled oats
½ cup rice flour
1¼ cups non-dairy milk
1 tablespoon canola oil
2 eggs, beaten
1 tablespoon honey
1 teaspoon baking powder
1 pinch of salt

Combine non-dairy milk, rolled oats, and rice flour, and set aside for several minutes. Then add the canola oil, eggs, honey, baking powder, and salt, mixing as you add each ingredient. Cook over medium heat on lightly oiled surface. Serve with maple syrup or fresh fruit preserves.

Corn Muffins

Serves 8 to 10

2 tablespoons canola oil
3 tablespoons honey
2 eggs, beaten
2 cups non-dairy milk, vanilla
2 cups corn meal
½ cup rice flour
½ teaspoon salt
1 teaspoon baking powder
½ teaspoon baking soda

Combine oil, honey, eggs, and non-dairy milk, and set aside. Combine corn meal, rice flour, salt, baking powder, and baking soda, and mix with wet ingredients until batter is smooth. Spoon into well-oiled muffin tins and bake about 20 minutes at 425°. Delicious with fresh flax oil, blackberry preserves, or raw almond butter.

Corn Waffles

Serves 4 to 6

3 eggs
¼ cup safflower oil
2 tablespoons honey
4 heaping tablespoons whey
2 cups water
1 teaspoon soda (level)
2 teaspoons baking soda (level)
1 teaspoon salt
1 cup corn flour
½ cup wheat flour
½ cup barley flour

Separate eggs, beat whites stiff. Beat yolks until creamy, then add sugar and oil. Add liquid ingredients. Mix dry ingredients and add to liquid mixture. Fold in egg whites. Prepare as waffles or hotcakes.

SPREADS

Tofu and Sesame-Butter Spread

Makes 1½ cups

½ cup tofu, drained
1 cup raw sesame butter
1 to 2 tablespoons honey

Blend all ingredients in a blender or food processor.

Sesame-Almond Butter

Makes 1½ cups

¼ cup soft tofu, drained
¼ cup raw sesame butter
6 tablespoons raw almond butter
¼ cup honey

Combine all ingredients in a blender.

Apple-Spice Butter

Makes 2 cups

1 pound apples, peeled, quartered,
   and cored
¼ to ½ cup water
½ teaspoon cinnamon
⅛ teaspoon cloves
¼ teaspoon ginger
2 tablespoons honey

Cook apples in water and cook for 5 to 10 minutes or until soft. Add spices and honey to pan. Stir to mix. Cool. Blend in blender or food processor until smooth.

Banana with Almond Butter

Serves 1

1 banana
2 tablespoons raw almond butter

Cut banana lengthwise in half. Cut each piece in half so that the banana is in four sections. Spread with almond butter.

Fresh Applesauce

Makes 2⅓ cups

½ cup fresh apple juice
2½ apples
½ teaspoon cinnamon

Peel apples and cut into quarters. Combine all ingredients in blender. Blend until smooth.

Lunch and Dinner

SOUPS

Tomato Soup
Serves 8

2 garlic cloves, minced
1 onion, chopped
2 tablespoons olive oil
4 tomatoes, chopped
8 cups canned tomatoes, chopped,
   low sodium, plus liquid

Cook garlic and onions in olive oil until soft. Transfer to large pot. Add canned and fresh tomatoes. Cover pot and cook on low heat for one hour.

High-Calcium Fish Stock
Makes 1 gallon

4 pounds white fish bones and
   heads
1 gallon water
1 onion, quartered
1 shallot
1 carrot
1 celery stalk
¼ cup chopped mushrooms
1 tablespoon peppercorns
1 cup dry white table wine
2 teaspoons vinegar

Place the fish bones and heads in an 8-quart stock pot; add the wine, vinegar, and water and bring very slowly to a boil. Remove the surface foam. Cut up the vegetables and add to the stock pot. Turn the heat down and simmer for 30 minutes. Strain the finished stock.

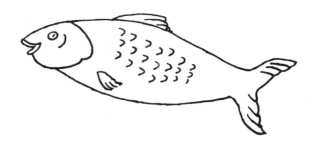

Vegetable Soup

Serves 4 to 6

1 onion, chopped
1 stalk celery, chopped
1 turnip, chopped
½ leek, chopped
2 carrots, chopped
¼ bunch parsley, chopped
5 mushrooms, sliced
½ tablespoon fennel
1 bay leaf
½ tablespoon thyme
1½ quarts water

Place all ingredients in a pot. Cover with water. Bring to a boil, then turn heat to low. Cook for 2 hours. Pour the soup into individual serving dishes.

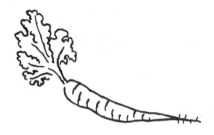

Lentil Soup

Serves 4

1 cup lentils
½ onion, chopped
½ cup carrots, chopped
1 to 1½ quarts water
1 teaspoon brown rice miso

Wash lentils. Put lentils, onion, carrots, water, and miso in a pot. Bring to a boil, then turn heat to low, cover pot and simmer for 45 minutes, or until lentils are soft.

Split Pea Soup

Serves 4

1 cup split peas
½ onion, chopped
1 small carrot, sliced
1 quart water
¼ teaspoon sea salt

Wash peas. Place peas, onion, and carrot in a pot. Add the water. Bring to a boil, then turn heat to low and cover pot. Cook for 45 minutes. Add sea salt and continue to cook until peas are soft. Soup may be cooled and then pureed in a blender if you prefer a creamy texture.

Beet Borscht

Serves 6 to 8

3 pints water
1 pint raw grated beets
⅓ cup honey
⅓ cup lemon juice

Bring water to a boil. Grate beets. Place beets in heavy kettle or earthen jar. Pour boiling water over beets and let stand overnight. Strain, add honey and lemon to the liquid. Serve chilled.

Potassium Broth

Serves 8 to 10

3 cups water
1 cup sliced carrots
1 cup sliced broccoli
1 cup sliced squash (zucchini
   or summer squash)
½ cup mushrooms
½ cup celery
2 tablespoons diced parsley
8 fresh tomatoes
1 onion, diced
2 garlic cloves, diced
¼ to 1 teaspoon basil (to taste)

Liquify tomatoes in a blender. Combine all ingredients in soup pot and bring to a boil for 30 minutes. Simmer for 30 minutes. Strain and serve.

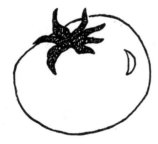

SALADS

Carrot-Raisin Salad
Serves 2

3 carrots
½ cup raisins
1 tablespoon mayonnaise
1 tablespoon cider vinegar

Peel and grate carrots. Mix shredded carrots and raisins with mayonnaise and cider vinegar.

Cabbage Slaw
Serves 4

1 cup red cabbage
3 cups green cabbage
1½ teaspoons caraway seeds
½ teaspoon poppy seeds
½ teaspoon celery seeds
½ teaspoon dill

Finely shred cabbage. Place in ice water 10 to 15 minutes, then drain. Crush or grind the seeds and add to shredded cabbage. Serve with favorite dressing.

Waldorf Salad

Serves 8

⅛ cup fresh lemon juice
6 crunchy apples
3 celery stalks, chopped
½ cup walnuts, chopped
8 lettuce leaves
4 tablespoons honey

Cut apples into eight pieces and sprinkle with lemon juice to keep color from turning brown. Combine the apples, celery, and walnuts. Drizzle this mixture with honey and toss gently. Spoon mixture onto lettuce leaves and serve.

Mixed Green Salad

Serves 4 to 6

1 head green or red leaf lettuce
1 large tomato, cut into wedges
½ cucumber, sliced
2 green onions, chopped
1 carrot, sliced
4 radishes, sliced
1 avocado, sliced
¼ cup sunflower seeds

Combine all ingredients in a large salad bowl. Serve with your favorite dressing.

Romaine Salad

Serves 4

1 head romaine lettuce
⅛ head red cabbage, chopped
4 radishes, sliced
1 small carrot, grated
oil and vinegar to taste

Combine all ingredients in a bowl and toss with oil and vinegar.

Potato Salad

Serves 6

8 red potatoes, medium
1 cup celery, chopped
½ cup parsley, finely chopped
¾ cup onions, chopped

Steam potatoes for approximately 45 minutes. Cool and cube. Combine celery, parsley, and onions with potatoes, mix thoroughly. Add a small amount of your favorite dressing. Both vinaigrette and mayonnaise are delicious on potato salad.

Watercress Salad

Serves 4

2 bunches watercress
6 ounces fresh bean sprouts
2 teaspoons scallions, finely
    chopped
½ tablespoon sunflower seeds
vinaigrette dressing

Wash watercress. Remove the large stems and place the rest in a bowl. Add bean sprouts and scallions. Toss the salad. Add the sunflower seeds and vinaigrette dressing and toss again. Serve immediately.

Calcium Salad

Serves 6

1 head romaine lettuce
1 avocado, sliced
¾ cup turnips, sliced
¾ cup celery, diced
¾ cup green onions, sliced
¾ cup watercress
¾ cup carrots, grated

Combine all ingredients in a large salad bowl and toss lightly. Serve with your favorite low-calorie French dressing.

Tomato Salad with Green Beans

Serves 4

1 pound green beans
1 tomato, chopped
3 teaspoons green onions, minced
1 garlic clove, minced
¼ teaspoon black pepper
1 teaspoon oregano

Steam green beans for 6 minutes. Texture should be crisp. Combine all ingredients in a large salad bowl. Dress with your favorite vinaigrette dressing.

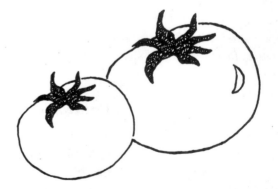

Guacamole Dip

Serves 4

2 ripe avocados
2 tablespoons lemon juice
1 green onion, diced
1 garlic clove, minced
1 tomato, chopped
2 carrots, sliced cocktail size
1 red pepper, sliced
4 large mushrooms, sliced

Peel the avocados, place them in a bowl and mash them with a fork. Add the lemon juice, onion, garlic, and tomato, stirring well. Chill and serve as a dip for the carrots, peppers, and mushrooms.

SANDWICHES

Healthy Sandwiches

Serves 1

2 pieces bread (rye, millet, rice,
 mixed whole grain, pita)
2 leaves lettuce
2 slices tomato
⅛ cup sprouts (optional)
½ cup sandwich spread (avocado,
 eggplant, tuna, vegetarian,
 raw almond butter, or jam)

Arrange lettuce, tomato, and sprouts on 1 slice of bread. Add sandwich spread to other slice. Combine and serve.

Avocado Sandwich Spread

Serves 2 to 4

1 avocado, mashed
2 tablespoons mayonnaise
½ teaspoon lemon juice
½ teaspoon paprika

Peel and mash avocado in bowl with fork. Add remaining ingredients and mix thoroughly. Serve on thin slices of bread or rye crackers.

Tuna Sandwich Filling

Serves 4

6 ounces canned tuna in water,
  drained
2 teaspoons mayonnaise
2 teaspoons green onions
2 tablespoons celery, chopped

Combine all ingredients in a bowl and mix thoroughly. Serve on bread or crackers.

Eggplant Sandwich Spread

Serves 4

1 eggplant, medium
1 onion, finely chopped
1 cup celery, diced
1 lemon, juiced
2 tablespoons olive oil
¼ cup black olives, chopped
1 garlic clove, minced

Bake eggplant at 350° F until soft. Then remove skin and mash to a smooth texture. Combine all other ingredients, letting stand at least 5 minutes. Combine eggplant with other ingredients, mix thoroughly. Chill and serve on bread or crackers.

Vegetarian Sandwich Filling

Serves 1

4 slices avocado
4 thin slices carrot
2 slices red onion
2 slices tomato

Combine in sandwich and serve.

Almond Butter and Jam

Serves 1

3 tablespoons raw almond butter
3 tablespoons no-sugar jam

Combine in sandwich and serve.

GRAINS, LEGUMES, STARCHES

Brown Rice
Serves 4

1 cup brown rice
2 cups cold water
½ teaspoon sea salt

Wash rice with cold water. Combine all ingredients in a cooking pot. Bring ingredients to a rapid boil. Turn flame to low, cover, and cook without stirring (about 25 to 35 minutes) until rice is soft. Resist the temptation to check before 20 minutes, because that lets out too much steam.

Kasha
Serves 4

1 cup kasha (buckwheat groats)
3¼ cups water
pinch salt

Bring ingredients to a boil, lower heat, and simmer for 25 minutes or until soft. The grains should be fluffy like rice. For breakfast, blend in blender with water till it is a "cream." Add almond milk, sesame milk, or sunflower milk; and cinnamon, apple butter, ginger, raisins, or berries.

Adzuki Beans
Serves 4

1 cup adzuki beans
4 cups water
¼ teaspoon sea salt

Wash beans. Place beans in a pot with the water and salt. Bring water to boil, cover and simmer for 2 hours or until beans are tender.

Baked Potato
Serves 4

4 russet or Idaho potatoes
1 tablespoon vegetable oil
2 tablespoons green onions,
   chopped

Preheat oven to 400° F. Wash the potatoes, rub them with vegetable oil, and bake for 45 to 60 minutes or until soft when pierced with a fork. Garnish with green onions.

VEGETABLES

Steamed Artichokes
Serves 4

4 artichokes

Trim the artichokes. Place them in a steamer with sufficient water to steam for 45 minutes. Remove from steamer and serve hot or cold. Use mayonnaise or your favorite vinaigrette.

Celery Julienne
Serves 4

6 stalks celery
2 tablespoons sweet red pepper, chopped

Cut the celery into small strips (like french fried potatoes). Steam for 15 to 20 minutes, or until tender. Drain and toss with red pepper.

Diced Carrots with Peas
Serves 4

1½ cups chicken stock
1 cup green peas
1 cup carrots, diced

Heat the chicken broth to boiling, then turn to low. Add the peas and carrots and simmer for 30 minutes or until vegetables are tender.

Cauliflower with Parsley
Serves 4

1 head medium cauliflower
3–4 tablespoons fresh parsley, finely chopped

Break the cauliflower into small flowerets. Steam 10 minutes or until tender. Toss with fresh parsley.

Broccoli with Lemon
Serves 4

1 pound broccoli
juice of ½ lemon

Cut the broccoli into small flowerets; steam for 12 minutes or until tender. Squeeze lemon juice over broccoli and serve.

Carrots Lark
Serves 4

12 small carrots, cleaned and sliced
4 tablespoons pecans, chopped
1 tablespoon maple syrup

Steam carrots until soft. Combine with pecans and drizzle with maple syrup.

Zucchini with Scallions
Serves 4

2 zucchini, medium, diced
2 teaspoons scallions, chopped
2 teaspoons safflower oil
½ garlic clove, minced
1 teaspoon dried basil
1 teaspoon oregano

Heat oil in frying pan on medium heat. Add all ingredients to frying pan. Cook until tender, stirring constantly.

Whipped Acorn Squash
Serves 4

2 acorn squash
2–3 ounces apple juice
pinch ground cinnamon

Peel and cut acorn squash into large pieces. Steam until tender. Place in food processor, add apple juice and cinnamon, and puree. You may also want to add water in small amounts until smooth and creamy.

SEEDS AND NUTS

Flax Cereal
Serves 1

6 tablespoons raw flax seeds
4 ounces apple juice
¼ teaspoon cinnamon

Take a coffee or seed grinder and grind the flax seeds to a powder. Put the ground flax seed into a cereal bowl and stir in the apple juice until the mixture thickens into a cereal-like consistency. Sprinkle cinnamon on top.

Flax Shakes
Serves 2

6 tablespoons raw flax seeds
1 whole banana, peeled
6 ounces apple juice
6 ounces water
1 tablespoon honey

Take a coffee or seed grinder and grind the flax seeds to a powder. Put the ground flax into a blender, add the remaining ingredients, and blend.

Flax Spread
Serves 2

6 tablespoons flax seeds
juice of half a lemon
½ teaspoon Bragg's liquid amino
    acids
2 tablespoons water

Take a coffee or seed grinder and grind the flax seeds to a powder. Put the ground flax seeds in a bowl, add the remaining ingredients, and mix into a paste. Use as a spread on rice cakes or rye crackers.

Hummus and Tahini (Sesame Butter)
Makes 3 cups

½ cup raw unhulled sesame seeds
1½ cups unsalted garbanzo beans,
    cooked
½ cup water
juice of one lemon
2 cloves garlic, minced
water, to taste

Take a coffee or seed grinder and grind the sesame seeds into a fine paste. Transfer to a blender. Add garbanzo beans, lemon juice, and garlic cloves. Blend until smooth, adding water until a dip consistency is achieved. Use as a dip for fresh vegetables like carrots and broccoli, or spread on rye bread.

FISH

Poached Salmon
Serves 4

4 fillets of salmon, 3 ounces each
1 cup water
1 lemon
1 tablespoon onion, diced
1 tablespoon carrot, diced
2 ounces low-sodium tomato juice

Combine the water and the juice of one lemon in skillet and heat. Place the salmon in the hot liquid and sprinkle with diced vegetables. Cover and poach for 6 to 8 minutes or until salmon flakes easily with a fork. Remove the fish and keep it warm. Add the tomato juice to the stock and reduce the liquid by one half. Cover the salmon with the sauce and serve hot.

Broiled Trout with Dill
Serves 4

2 fresh trout, about 8 ounces each
2 tablespoons lemon juice
chopped fresh dill (dried if fresh
  is unavailable)

Slice each trout in half and bone. This will make four fillets. Sprinkle the fillets with lemon juice and dill. Place the trout in a broiler pan. Broil for 5 or 6 minutes or until done.

Poached Halibut
Serves 4

4 flounder fillets, 3 ounces each
2 cups water
2 shallots, chopped
2 sprigs parsley
1 small stalk celery, chopped
1 bay leaf

Combine water, shallots, parsley, and bay leaf in a pot. Cover and simmer for 10 minutes. Strain. Gently add the flounder to the liquid. Cover the pot and simmer for 10 minutes or until fish is tender.

One-Dish Meals

Almond Tofu
Serves 4

¾ cup celery, finely chopped
½ cup water
1 teaspoon sesame or safflower oil
1 cup tofu, cubed
¼ cup blanched almonds
3 cups brown rice, cooked
tamari soy sauce

Sauté celery in water and oil over a low flame for 20 minutes or until tender. Add tofu and almonds and cook for 5 minutes. Transfer to a serving dish and toss with rice and tamari sauce to taste.

Tofu with Snow Peas
Serves 4

¾ cup tofu, cubed
1 cup snow peas, steamed
¼ cup water
1 teaspoon sesame or safflower oil
3 cups brown rice, cooked
tamari soy sauce

Combine tofu and snow peas in a large frying pan with water and oil. Cook over low flame for 5 minutes. (Add extra water to pan if needed.) Add rice to pan and mix. Heat for 5 minutes or until warm. Transfer to serving dish and toss with tamari soy sauce to taste.

Tacos
Serves 4

4 corn tortillas
1 pound pinto beans, cooked and
   pureed
½ avocado, thinly sliced
¼ yellow onion, finely chopped
6 tablespoons salsa
½ head red or romaine lettuce,
   chopped

Warm tortillas and beans in separate pans. Place tortillas on individual serving dishes and spread with beans. Garnish with avocado and onion, then cover each taco with lettuce and 1½ tablespoons of salsa.

Chop Suey

Serves 4

2 cups zucchini, thinly sliced
2 medium onions, sliced
1 cup bean sprouts
1 cup celery, thinly sliced
1 cup green onions
¼ cup olive oil
2 cups cooked brown rice

Put olive oil in pan and heat (medium). Add zucchini, onions, sprouts, celery, and green onions. Cover and sauté until vegetables are slightly tender. Do not overcook. Serve over brown rice.

Stuffed Peppers

Serves 6

6 green peppers
¾ cup celery, diced
1 cup onions, chopped
2 cups cooked brown rice
½ cup tomato juice (low-sodium)
¼ teaspoon sea salt
2 cups spaghetti sauce

Preheat over to 350° F. Scoop out peppers. Mix all other ingredients except spaghetti sauce. Fill peppers with mixture. Put peppers in baking dish. Pour spaghetti sauce over pepper and bake uncovered for 45 minutes. Serve hot.

Tofu-Wild Rice Salad

Serves 4

6 ounces tofu
2 cups cooked wild rice
3 scallions, chopped
¼ to ½ cup minced parsley
½ green pepper, minced
herbal oil and vinegar dressing

Cut tofu into bite-size pieces. Combine with all the other ingredients in a bowl. Mix with your favorite herbal oil and vinegar dressing to taste. Note: brown rice may be substituted for wild rice.

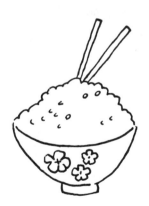

Tofu and Brown Rice

Serves 4

2 cups cooked brown rice
1 cup tofu, diced
1 green onion, diced
¼ cup raisins
1½ ounces blanched almonds
¼ cup peas, cooked
¼ cup green pepper
¼ cup celery

Combine all ingredients in a bowl. The salad may be dressed with a vinaigrette dressing or with a dressing made by combining 1½ tablespoons seasoned rice wine vinegar, ½ teaspoon Worcestershire sauce, and 2½ tablespoons mayonnaise.

Desserts

High-Calcium Pound Cake

Serves 8

2½ cups rice flour
½ teaspoon baking soda
1½ teaspoons baking powder
½ teaspoon sea salt
1 teaspoon vanilla
⅓ cup honey
½ cup corn oil
2 eggs
1 cup nut or sesame milk
1,500 mg calcium powder

Preheat oven to 350° F. Sift together flour, baking soda, baking powder, calcium, and salt. Mix corn oil, honey, and vanilla together. Separate eggs. Beat the yolks and add to corn oil, honey, and vanilla mixture. Slowly add sifted ingredients to egg mixture with the nut or sesame milk. Beat egg whites until stiff peaks form and fold them into the dough. Place dough in well-greased pan and bake for 30 to 40 minutes or until a knife inserted in center of cake is clean when removed.

High-Calcium Cashew Ice Milk

Serves 6 to 8

½ cup water
agar-agar flakes (poured to the 3-
    ounce mark in a measuring cup)
2 cups apple juice
2 egg yolks
1 cup cashew milk
2 tablespoons honey
½ teaspoon vanilla
500 mg liquid calcium

Agar-agar is a gelatin made from seaweed. It is used as a thickening agent and can be found in most health food stores.

Combine agar-agar with water and cook over a low flame until it dissolves. Combine agar-agar, apple juice, cashew milk, vanilla, calcium, and honey. Combine egg yolks with a few teaspoons of the mixture. Add this to the rest of the mixture. Cook at low heat until thickened, stirring continuously. Pour mixture into individual serving bowls and freeze.

Banana and Sesame Butter

Serves 2

2 bananas, ripened
3 tablespoons raw sesame butter
½ teaspoon honey

Mash bananas in bowl and slowly blend in raw sesame butter and honey. This makes a highly nutritious dessert for menopausal women.

Apple-Tofu Custard

Serves 2

4 ounces soft tofu
1 apple, red Delicious
1 banana, ripened
½ teaspoon honey

Combine tofu, apple, banana, and honey in blender and mix until a custard-like consistency is achieved.

Baked Bananas

Serves 4

4 bananas
1 tablespoon lemon juice
2 tablespoons honey

Peel and slice bananas in half lengthwise. Place halves in well-oiled baking dish. Sprinkle with lemon juice and drizzle with honey. Put in cold oven set to 400° F. When juice begins to bubble, turn off heat. Leave in oven to finish baking on retained heat.

Persimmon Banana Treat

Serves 4

4 bananas
3 persimmons, ripe
2 tablespoons honey
½ cup coconut

Remove skin of persimmons and mash. Peel and slice bananas very thin. In each serving dish, alternate layers of banana and persimmon. Sprinkle with honey and cover with fine coconut. Chill and serve.

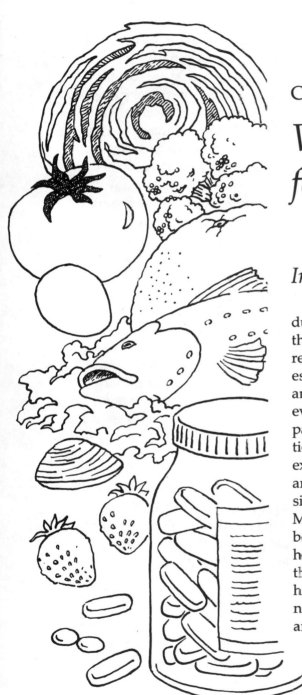

CHAPTER 9

Vitamins and Minerals for Menopause

Introduction

Optimal intake of vitamins and minerals is extremely important during the menopause and postmenopausal years. As women lose their hormonal support and the body's metabolism and chemical reactions become less efficient with age, an adequate intake of essential building blocks is critical to support repair, regeneration, and maintenance of our cells. A good supplement program can even help to relieve and prevent many of the symptoms of menopause. This is much more desirable than taking strong medications, which can have dangerous or deleterious side effects. For example, antidepressants are often given for menopause fatigue and depression, when medical studies of potassium and magnesium aspartate show dramatic results in improving energy levels. Many women do not want to take hormones for hot flashes because of their fear of the side effects. Other women cannot use hormones for medical reasons, such as breast or uterine cancer. For these women, the use of nutritional supplements may be quite helpful. Many medical studies show that vitamin E and bioflavonoids can help relieve menopause symptoms greatly. Women who are on hormonal therapy should also consider using a well-planned program of nutritional supplements to maintain optimal health.

As you read this chapter you will learn about the incredibly beneficial effects that nutrition can have on all menopause symptoms, including bleeding problems, hot flashes, vaginal and bladder changes, depression, fatigue, insomnia, anxiety, and osteoporosis. Nutrients are also essential in helping to prevent diseases of the female reproductive tract, thyroid problems, and many health problems associated with old age, such as heart disease and diabetes mellitus. In fact, poor or inadequate nutrition may cause these problems or contribute greatly to their onset. I consider a well-balanced menopause vitamin and mineral supplement program to be absolutely essential for any woman in mid-life and beyond. This is supported by hundreds of medical studies that have been done at many university centers and hospitals. For those wanting more technical information I have included at the end of this chapter a selected bibliography of more than one hundred medical studies on menopause and other problems related to aging.

Supplemental vitamins and minerals should not be used, however, as an excuse to continue poor dietary habits. They should be taken along with a low-stress nutritious diet to maintain optimal health. If you have particular health problems, it is important to make sure that both your diet and supplement program meet your body's needs for the extra nutrients that you require. For example, if you have a tendency toward heavy bleeding in the year or two preceding menopause, extra iron, bioflavonoids, and vitamin C are important. Your diet should include foods high in these nutrients, such as liver, beet greens, and plenty of fruit. If you have a family history of osteoporosis, be sure to eat plenty of beans, leafy green vegetables, and salmon, along with calcium supplements to help prevent osteoporosis. The next section will discuss the nutrients that help to relieve the specific health problems related to menopause.

Vitamins and Minerals for Menopause

Vitamin A. Vitamin A is necessary for the growth and support of the skin, mucous membranes, and eyes. Deficiency of vitamin A causes night blindness, rough, scaly skin, fatigue, and an increased susceptibility to infections. Interestingly enough, medical studies have shown that low vitamin A intake can also put a woman at higher risk of heavy menstrual bleeding, abnormal Pap smears, and cervical cancer. A lack of adequate vitamin A can predispose a woman to skin conditions related to the aging process, such as vulvar leukoplakia and senile keratosis. Both of these conditions can precede the onset of skin cancer. Vitamin A has also been used successfully to treat noncancerous breast lumps at the University of Montreal Medical School.

Vitamin B-Complex. The B-complex vitamins are usually found together in foods such as beans, whole grains, and liver. Several of the B vitamins are particularly important for supplemental menopause-related problems. Vitamin B6 should be taken if you are using estrogen replacement therapy. Hormonal therapy leads to a deficiency in this vitamin. Folic acid is important in helping to prevent cervical dysplasia (which can be a precursor to cervical cancer). It is important, however, to have an adequate intake of all the eleven vitamin B factors. The whole complex works together to perform important metabolic functions, including glucose metabolism, inactivation of estrogen by the liver, and stabilization of brain chemistry. The B-complex vitamins are water-soluble. The emotional stress related to menopause can cause the loss of the B vitamins from the body. Fatigue and irritability can be the result.

My recommended therapeutic dosages for menopause (menopause RDA) for some of the important B vitamins are:

Thiamin (vitamin B1)	50 mg
Riboflavin (vitamin B2)	50 mg
Niacin (vitamin B3)	50 mg
Biotin	30 mcg
Pantothenic acid (vitamin B5)	50 mg
Pyridoxine (vitamin B6)	30 mg
Para-aminobenzoic acid	50 mg
Choline	50 mg
Inositol	50 mg
Cyanocobalamin (vitamin B12)	50 mcg
Folic acid	400 mg

Vitamin C. Vitamin C is found abundantly in nature. Many fruits and vegetables as well as some meats contain high levels of vitamin C. A low vitamin C intake has been found to predispose women to cervical dysplasia and excessive menstrual bleeding (menorrhagia).

The diet of women with early-stage cervical cancer has been compared to those of healthy controls in medical research studies. The women with cervical cancer were found to have a diet much lower in foods containing vitamin C. Vitamin C helps to maintain collagen and heal wounds and burns. It is an important anti-stress vitamin which helps to fight infections and allergies. Large amounts of vitamin C are found in the adrenal gland where it is used for adrenal cortical hormone synthesis.

Bioflavonoids. This is one of the most important nutrients for women with menopause. In fact, along with vitamin E, it could be called the "menopause vitamin." Bioflavonoids have chemical activity similar to estrogen and can be used as an estrogen substitute. Clinical studies have shown the remarkable ability of bioflavonoids to control hot flashes and the psychological symptoms of menopause. Many women with anxiety, irritability, and menopause-related mood swings noted considerable relief of their symptoms. Unlike estrogen therapy, no harmful side effects have been noted with bioflavonoid therapy. Bioflavonoids have also shown dramatic results in relieving heavy menstrual bleeding due to their ability to strengthen the capillary walls. They were given in the medical studies along with vitamin C. Bioflavonoids can be found abundantly in citrus fruits, especially in the pulp and the white of the rind.

Vitamin D. Many medical studies have demonstrated the importance of vitamin D for the prevention of osteoporosis. It aids in the absorption of calcium from the intestinal tract and in the assimilation of phosphorus. Adequate vitamin D is essential to maintain strong, sturdy bones through and beyond the menopause period. It is a fat-soluble vitamin that can either be ingested through food intake or acquired through exposure to sunlight. A vitamin D precursor on the skin surface is converted to vitamin D through the action of sunlight.

Vitamin E. Vitamin E has been studied for the past forty years for its usefulness in relieving a number of female complaints. Along with bioflavonoids, it can act as an estrogen substitute, relieving hot flashes and the psychological symptoms of menopause. This has been demonstrated in a number of very interesting medical studies. Research studies have also demonstrated the ability of vitamin E to relieve atrophic vaginitis, which can be a real blessing for the many women who suffer from vaginal soreness, dryness, and pain in intercourse. If you suffer from this problem, you might take vitamin E by mouth and also open a capsule and apply the oil directly to your vaginal tissue. Vitamin E is really an essential part of the supplemental program for women during the menopause years. Vitamin E has also been studied for its ability to reduce breast cysts and premenstrual tension, and to maintain thyroid function. Besides its usefulness for specific female complaints, research studies suggest that it is a helpful treatment for many skin conditions, osteoarthritis, and heart disease.

Vitamin E is an important antioxidant and protects the cells from the destructive effects of many environmental chemicals that can react with the polyunsaturated fats in the cell membranes. Oxidation of the cell can accelerate the aging process as well as the onset of many diseases. Vitamin E is found most abundantly in vegetable oils, nuts, and seeds, as well as in some fruits and vegetables.

Calcium. Calcium is absolutely vital for strong and healthy bones. While the recommended daily allowance for calcium is 800 mg per day for adults, most women during the menopause years only get half of what they need from their diet. Some women may have difficulty absorbing calcium from their intestinal tract due to lack of necessary enzymes, especially if they depend on dairy sources of calcium. These dairy sources become increasingly difficult to digest with age. Because of the hormonal changes that occur around the time of menopause, 1,000 to 1,200 mg of calcium per day is absolutely necessary to prevent osteoporosis. To ensure adequate intake, a calcium supplement should be used in addition to a diet rich in legumes, green leafy vegetables, fish, seeds, and nuts. Calcium is also useful in helping to control high blood pressure and elevated blood fats, which can predispose you to heart disease.

Magnesium. Magnesium is an important mineral found in the bone, and adequate intake is necessary along with calcium and vitamin D for bone health. It has been studied, along with potassium, as an effective therapy for the treatment of menopause fatigue. Women who complain of low energy and lack of vitality with menopause should be sure to take a magnesium supplement of 400 mg along with a magnesium-rich diet. Many of the foods high in calcium are also rich in magnesium. See the food chart for a list of the specific foods. Magnesium helps to normalize glucose metabolism and to stabilize moods by its effect on brain chemistry. It is also important to have adequate magnesium levels for the prevention of diabetes mellitus and coronary artery disease.

Potassium. Potassium is an essential mineral that constitutes five percent of the body's total mineral content. It is necessary for normal muscle contraction and heartbeat, and helps to preserve the acid-base balance of the body in a healthy range. It also helps to regulate the fluid balance of the body. Potassium, along with magnesium, has been found to relieve menopause fatigue in medical studies. Women using potassium and magnesium aspartate supplements reported much greater energy levels than without the addition of the minerals. Good sources of potassium include bananas, citrus fruits, potatoes, and nuts.

Iron Women who suffer from heavy menstrual bleeding require supplemental iron intake. In fact, some medical studies have found that supplemental iron actually relieves the problem, suggesting that inadequate iron intake may be a cause of menorrhagia. Iron is absorbed better if taken with vitamin C. Iron is an essential component of blood: it combines with protein and copper in making hemoglobin, the pigment of the red blood cells. Iron can be found in liver, molasses, and yeast.

Iodine. Iodine is essential for the development and functioning of the thyroid gland. It is a necessary part of thyroxine, the principal hormone produced by the thyroid gland. Several medical studies suggest that it plays a role in maintaining healthy breast tissue and preventing breast disease. Adequate iodine intake is necessary for stimulating the body's metabolism, promoting growth and development, and regulating the body's energy production. Iodine is found in sea plants and animals. Fish, seaweed, and shellfish, all excellent sources of iodine, absorb it from sea water. People who live in landlocked areas can be prone to iodine deficiency which can cause goiter and hypothyroidism. Iodine supplements may be easily obtained through using dulse or kelp tablets.

Essential Fatty Acids for Menopause

Essential fatty acids are very important nutrients for women in the menopause years. Because of the important role that they play in maintaining optimal health I am including them in the vitamin and mineral chapter. Essential fatty acids consist of two types of special fats called linoleic acid (Omega-6 Family) and linolenic acid (Omega-3 Family). These fats can not be made by the body and must be supplied daily in your diet from either foods or supplements. While these essential fatty acids supply stored energy in the form of calories, they also perform many other important functions in the body. Essential fatty acids are important components of the membrane structure of all the cells of the body. They are also required for normal development and function of the brain, eyes, inner ear, adrenal glands, and reproductive tract. The essential oils are also necessary for the synthesis of prostaglandins type I and III. These prostaglandins are hormone-like chemicals that help to decrease the risk of heart disease by regulating blood pressure and platelet stickiness. Protaglandins type I and III also decrease inflammation, boost immune function, decrease menstrual cramps, and help to reduce PMS symptoms. In fact, one essential fat called evening primrose oil is being tested in the United States and England for its beneficial effects on PMS and menstrual cramps. Essential oils are particularly important to menopausal women because the deficiency of these oils is responsible in part for the drying of the skin, hair, vaginal tissues, and other mucous membranes that occurs with menopause. Along with vitamin E, which also benefits the skin and vaginal tissues, I have used essential oils extensively in my nutritional programs for women. Many of my patients have noted a definite improvement in vaginal lubrication and moister, softer skin with the use of my program. I have also had several patients with very small breasts note an increase in their breast size with the use of the essential oils. They were obviously delighted as this gave them a more balanced figure.

The best sources of both essential fatty acids (linoleic and linolenic acids) are flax seeds and pumpkin seeds. Both the seeds and their pressed oils should be used absolutely fresh and unspoiled. Because these oils become rancid very easily when exposed to light and air (oxygen), they need to be packed in special opaque containers and kept in the refrigerator. Fresh flax seed oil is my special favorite. Good-quality flax seed oil is available from both Spectrum Marketing, Inc., of Petaluma, California, and Bio-San in Fountain Hills, Arizona. Both brands are now available in health food stores. Flax seed oil is golden, rich, and delicious. It is extremely high in linoleic and linolenic acid (which comprise approximately 80% of its total content). Flax seed oil has the most wonderful flavor and can be used as a butter replacement on foods such as mashed potatoes, air-popped popcorn, steamed broccoli, cauliflower, carrots, and bread. Flax seed oil (and all other essential oils) should never be heated or used in cooking as it effects the special chemical properties of these oils. These oils should always be added to foods that are already cooked as a form of flavoring at the end. Pumpkin seed oil has a deep green color and spicy flavor. It is probably more difficult to find than flax seed oil. A good source of this oil can be obtained by eating fresh raw pumpkin seeds. They can be purchased from your local health food store and should be kept refrigerated because they are highly perishable. Both flax seed oil and pumpkin seed oil can be used in capsule form.

Linolenic acid (Omega-3 Family) is also found in abundance in fish oils. The best sources are cold-water, high-fat fish such as salmon, tuna, rainbow trout, mackerel, and eel. Linoleic acid (Omega-6 Family) is found in seeds and seed oils. Good sources include safflower oil, sunflower oil, corn oil, sesame seed oil, and wheat germ oil. Many women prefer to use raw fresh sesame seeds, sunflower seeds, and wheat germ to obtain the oils. The average healthy adult requires only four teaspoons per day of the essential oils in their diet. However, menopausal women with extremely dry skin, hair, and vaginal tissues may have a real deficiency of these oils and need up to two to three tablespoons per day until their symptoms improve. As I mentioned earlier, be sure to use these oils along with vitamin E for optimal results. I recommend that women during the menopause years use a combination of the following fatty acids.

Essential Oil Formula: Flax Oil
Borage Oil
Wheat Germ Oil
Fish Oil (Omega 3)
Vitamin E

Food Sources of Vitamin A

Vegetables	Fruits	Meats, Poultry, Fish, Seafood
carrot	apricot	
carrot juice	avocado	crab
collard greens	mango	halibut
dandelion greens	cantaloupe	liver—all types
green onions	papaya	mackerel
kale	peach	salmon
parsley	persimmon	swordfish
spinach		
sweet potato		
turnip greens		
winter squash		

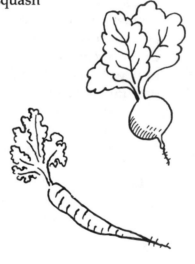

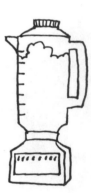

Food Sources of Vitamin C

Vegetables

asparagus
black-eyed peas
broccoli
brussels sprouts
cabbage
cauliflower
collards
green onions
green peas
kale
kohlrabi
parsley
potato
rutabaga
sweet pepper
sweet potato
tomato
turnips

Fruits

blackberries
black currants
cantaloupe melon
elderberries
grapefruit
grapefruit juice
guava
kiwi fruit
mango
orange
orange juice
pineapple
raspberries
strawberries
tangerine

Meats, Poultry, Fish, Seafood

liver—all types
pheasant
quail
salmon

Food Sources of Vitamin E

Vegetables

asparagus
cucumber
green peas
kale

Meats, Poultry, Fish, Seafood

haddock
herring
mackerel
lamb
liver—all types

Grains

brown rice
millet

Nuts and Seeds

almonds
Brazil nuts
hazelnuts
peanuts

Oils

corn oil
peanut oil
safflower oil
sesame oil
soybean oil
wheat germ oil

Fruits

mango

Food Sources of Calcium

Vegetables

artichoke
black beans
black-eyed peas
beet greens
broccoli
brussels sprouts
cabbage
collards
eggplant
garbanzo beans
green beans
green onions
kale
kidney beans
leeks
lentils
parsley
parsnips
pinto beans
rutabaga
soybeans
spinach
turnips
watercress

Grains

bran
brown rice
bulgar
millet

Meats, Poultry, Fish, Seafood

abalone
beef
bluefish
carp
cod
crab
haddock
herring
lamb
lobster
oysters
perch
salmon
shrimp
venison

Fruits

blackberries
black currants
boysenberries
orange
papaya
pineapple juice
prune
raisins
rhubarb
tangerine juice

Food Sources of Magnesium

Vegetables

artichoke
black-eyed peas
carrot juice
corn
green peas
leeks
lima beans
okra
parsnips
potato
soybean sprouts
spinach
squash
yams

Nuts and Seeds

almonds
Brazil nuts
hazelnuts
peanuts
pistachios
pumpkin seeds
sesame seeds
walnuts

Grains

millet
rice, brown and wild

Meat, Poultry, Fish, Seafood

beef
carp
clams
cod
chicken
crab
duck
haddock
herring
lamb
lobster
mackerel
oysters
salmon
shrimp
snapper
turkey

Fruits

avocado
banana
grapefruit juice
papaya
pineapple juice
prune
raisins

Nutrients that Help Menopause and Other Age-Related Problems

Vitamins and Minerals:	Benefits:
Vitamin A	Menorrhagia, benign breast disease, cervical dysplasia and cancer, vulvar leukoplakia, senile keratosis, other skin conditions
Folic Acid	Cervical dysplasia, osteoporosis, post-menopausal homocysteinemia, diabetes mellitus, nervous system
Vitamin B_3 (Niacin)	Hyperlipidemia, hypoglycemia
Vitamin B_6	Estrogen replacement therapy deficiency, cancer of the cervix, diabetes mellitus
Vitamin B_{12}	Fatigue, diabetes mellitus
Lecithin	Nervous system
Inositol	Nervous system
Vitamin C	Menorrhagia, cervical dysplasia, chloasma, pigmented contact dermatitis
Vitamin D	Osteoporosis
Vitamin E	Hot flashes, psychological symptoms of menopause, diabetic vulvovaginitis, mammary dysplasia, hypothyroidism, chloasma, pigmented contact dermatitis, other skin conditions, atherosclerosis, osteoarthritis
Calcium	Osteoporosis, hyperlipidemia, hypertension
Magnesium	Osteoporosis, menopausal fatigue, diabetes mellitus, coronary artery disease
Potassium	Menopausal fatigue, heart disease, hypertension

Zinc	Osteoporosis
Iron	Menorrhagia
Iodine	Mammary dysplasia, hypothyroidism
Chromium	Hypoglycemia
Selenium	Fibrocystic breast disease, breast cancer
Manganese	Cerebral artery disease

Menopause Symptoms and Nutrients that Help Relieve Them

Symptoms:	Nutrients:
Menorrhagia	Vitamin A Bioflavonoids Vitamin C Iron
Hot flashes	Bioflavonoids Vitamin E
Psychological symptoms, fatigue	Potassium Magnesium Vitamin B_{12}
Psychological symptoms, anxiety and irritability	Vitamin B Complex Bioflavonoids
Atrophic vaginitis	Vitamin E Bioflavonoids
Osteoporosis	Calcium Magnesium Vitamin D Zinc Folic Acid

Fibrocystic disease of the breast	Vitamin A
	Vitamin E
	Iodine
Breast cancer	Selenium
Hypothyroidism	Iodine
Cervical dysplasia and cancer	Vitamin A
	Folic Acid
	Vitamin C
	Vitamin B_6

Vitamin and Mineral Supplements for Women with Menopause

As we have already discussed, good dietary habits are crucial for control of menopause symptoms. For many women, however, the use of a nutritional supplement is important in order to achieve high levels of certain essential nutrients. I have formulated a vitamin-and-mineral supplement based on a review of forty years of medical research in this field. This supplement is unlike most of those that are commercially available because the levels of nutrients are specific for women in the menopause years, and they provide optimal nutrition for women concerned with health problems related to the aging process. I have found these nutrients to be very helpful to my patients. This supplement is available by mail order (see coupon at the back of the book). You can also put the supplement together yourself. The ingredients are listed at the end of this section. If you have specific questions about nutritional supplementation, be sure to consult your physician.

Optimal Nutritional Supplementation for Menopause

Beta carotene (Pro Vitamin A)	5,000 I.U.	Choline	50 mg
Vitamin A	5,000 I.U.	Inositol	50 mg
Vitamin D	400 I.U.	Para-Aminobenzoic Acid	50 mg
Vitamin E (d-alpha tocopheryl acetate)	800 I.U.	Calcium (Calcium Citrate)	1200 mg
		Magnesium	320 mg
Vitamin C	1,000 mg	Iodine	150 mcg
Bioflavonoids	800 mg	Iron (Ferrous Fumarate)	27 mg
Rutin	200 mg	Copper	2 mg
Vitamin B_1	50 mg	Zinc	15 mg
Vitamin B_2	50 mg	Manganese	10 mg
Niacin (as niacinamide)	50 mg	Potassium (Potassium Aspartate)	100 mg
Vitamin B_6	30 mg	Selenium	25 mcg
Vitamin B_{12}	50 mcg	Chromium	100 mcg
Folic Acid	400 mcg	Bromelain	100 mg
Biotin	200 mcg	Papain	65 mg
Pantothenic Acid	50 mg	Boron	3 mg

Women with mild to moderate menopause symptoms can use this formula at half strength. Women with severe symptoms should use the full strength.

Suggested Reading
Books

Greenwood, S., M.D. *Menopause Naturally*. Volcano Press, 1989.

Hasslering, B., S. Greenwood, M.D., and M. Castleman. *The Medical Self-Care Book of Women's Health*. New York: Doubleday, 1987.

Hogladaroom, G., R. McCorkle, and N. Woods. *The Complete Book of Women's Health*. Englewood Cliffs, N.J.: Prentice-Hall, 1982.

Kirschmann, J., and L. Dunne. *Nutrition Almanac*. New York: McGraw-Hill, 1984.

Kutsky, R. *Vitamins and Hormones*. New York: Van Nostrand Reinhold, 1973.

Lark, S., M.D. *Premenstrual Syndrome Self Help Book*. Berkeley, Ca.: Celestial Arts, 1984.

Padus, E. *The Woman's Encyclopedia of Health and Natural Healing*. Emmaus, Pa.: Rodale Press, 1981.

Reuben, C., and J. Priestly. *Essential Supplements for Women*. New York: Perigree Books, 1988.

Articles

Abrams, A. A. 1965. "Use of Vitamin E in Chronic Cystic Mastitis." *New England Journal of Medicine* 272:1080.

Albanese, A. A., et al. 1973. "Effect of a Calcium Supplement on Serum Cholesterol, Calcium Phosphorus and Bone Density of Normal, Healthy Elderly Females." *Nutrition Report International* 8:119.

Albanese, A.A., et al. 1981. "Effects of Calcium Supplements and Estrogen Replacement Therapy on Bone Loss of Postmenopausal Women." *Nutrition Reports International* 24:404.

Anastasi, J., and M. Steiner. 1974. "Effect of Alpha-Tocopherol on Known Platelet Aggregation." Div. of Hematologic Research, The Memorial Hospital; Pawtucket and Brown University, RI.

Anderson, R. A., et al. "Chromium Supplementation of Humans with Hypoglycemia." USDA, Beltsville Human Nutrition Research Center, Beltsville, MD.

Anonymous. 1981. "Physical Activity and Supplements Slowed Bone Loss in Elderly Women." *Physician and Sports Medicine* 9(9):8.

Ant, M. 1954. "Diabetic Vulvovaginitis Treated with Vitamin E Suppositories." *American Journal of Obstetrics and Gynecology* 67:407.

Aquino, T. I., and B. A. Eskin. 1972. "Rat Breast Structure in Altered Iodine Metabolism." *Archives of Pathology* 94:280.

Ayres, S., and R. Mihan. 1975. "Vitamin E and Dermatology." *Cutis* 16:1017.

Band, P. R., et al. 1984. "Treatment of Benign Breast Disease with Vitamin A." *Preventive Medicine* 13:549.

Bargallo Sangiorgi, G., et al. 1983. "Serum Potassium Level, Red Blood Cell Potassium and Alterations of Repolarization Phase of EKG in Old Subjects." European Congress of Clinical Gerontology.

Barrie, M. M. O. 1937. "Effect of Vitamin E Deficiency on the Thyroid." 2:286.

Bierenbaum, M. L., et al. 1971. "Long Term Human Studies on the Lipid Effects of Oral Calcium." *Lipids* 7:202.

Block, M. T. January 1953. "Vitamin E in the Treatment of Diseases of the Skin." *Clinical Medicine* 31.

Bordoni, A., et al. January 1987. "Treatment of Premenstrual Syndrome with Essential Fatty Acids (Evening Primrose Oil)." *Journal of Clinical Medicine* 68(1):23.

Botez, et al. 1976. "Neurologic Disorders Responsive to Folic Acid Therapy." *CMA Journal* 115:217.

Boykin, L. S. 1976. "Iron Deficiency Anemia in Postmenopausal Women." *Journal of the American Geriatrics Society* 24:558.

Brattstrom, L. E., et al. 1985. "Folic Acid Responsive Postmenopausal Homocysteinemia." *Metabolism* 34:1073.

Brush, M. G. "Evening Primrose Oil in the Treatment of Premenstrual Syndrome." *Clinical Uses of Essential Fatty Acids*. Edited by D. F. Horrobin. Montreal, Eden Press, 1983.

Butterworth, C. E., et al. 1982. "Improvement in Cervical Dysplasia Associated with Folic Acid Therapy in Users of Oral Contraceptives." *American Journal of Clinical Nutrition* 35:73.

Chalmers, R. J. G., and S. Shuster. 1983. "Evening Primrose Seed Oil in Ichthyosis Vulgaris." *Lancet* 1:236.

Cheng, E.W., et al. 1955. "Estrogenic Activity of Some Naturally Occurring Isoflavones." *Annals of New York Academy of Sciences* 61(3):652.

Chow, B. F., and H. F. Stone. 1957. "The Relationship of Vitamin B12 to Carbohydrate Metabolism and Diabetes Mellitus." *The American Journal of Clinical Nutrition* 5:431.

Christy, C. J. 1945. "Vitamin E in Menopause: Preliminary Report of Experimental and Clinical Study." *American Journal of Obstetrics and Gynecology* 50:84.

Chu, E. W., and R. A. Malmgren. 1964. "An Inhibitory Effect of Vitamin A on the Induction of Tumors of Forestomach and Cervix in the Syrian Hamster by Carcinogenic Polycyclic Hydrocarbons." *Cancer Research* 25:884.

Clemetson, C. A. B., et al. 1962. "Capillary Strength and the Menstrual Cycle." *New York Academy of Sciences* 93(7):277.

Cobb, J. O. 1987. "Demystifying Menopause." *The Canadian Nurse* 8:17.

Cohen, J. D., and H. W. Rubin. 1960. "Functional Menorrhagia: Treatment with Bioflavonoids and Vitamin C." *Current Therapeutic Research* 2(11):539.

Cohen, L., and R. Kitzes. 1981. "Infrared Spectroscopy and Magnesium Content of Bone Mineral in Osteoporotic Women." 17:1123.

Cohn, S. H., et al. 1968. "High Calcium Diet and the Parameters of Calcium Metabolism in Osteoporosis." *The American Journal of Clinical Nutrition* 21:1246.

Coplan, H. M., and M. M. Sampson. 1934. "The Effects of a Deficiency of Iodine and Vitamin A on the Thyroid Gland of the Albino Rat." *The Journal of Nutrition* 9:469.

Cordova, C., et al. 1981. "Influence of Ascorbic Acid on Platelet Aggregation in vitro and in vivo." *Atherosclerosis* 41:15.

Corson, S. L., and V. G. Upton. 1982. "The Perimenopause: Physiologic Correlates and Clinical Management." *Journal of Reproductive Medicine* 27:1.

Cutick, R. 1984. "Special Needs of Perimenopausal and Menopausal Women." *Journal of Obstetric and Gynecologic Nursing* 3:685.

Davis, R. E., et al. 1976. "Serum Pyridoxal and Folate Concentrations in Diabetes." *Pathology* 6:151.

Dublin, W. B., and E. M. Hazen. January 1948. "The Relation of Keratosis Seborrheica and Keratosis Senilis to Vitamin A Deficiency." *Archives of Dermatology* 178.

Ellis, F. R., and S. Nasser. 1973. "A Pilot Study of Vitamin B12 in the Treatment of Tiredness." *Journal of Nutrition* 30:277.

Elwood, J. C., et al. 1982. "Effect of High Chromium Brewer's Yeast on Human Serum Lipids." *Journal of the American College of Nutrition.* 1:263.

Eskin, E. A., et al. 1967. "Mammary Gland Dysplasia and Iodine Deficiency." *Journal of the American Medical Association* 200:115.

Ferguson, H. E. 1948. "The Use of Vitamin E in Menopausal Syndrome." *Virginia Medical Monthly* 9:447.

Finkler, R. S. 1949. "The Effect of Vitamin E in the Menopause." *Journal of Clinical Endocrinology* 9:89.

Formica, P. E. 1962. "The Housewife Syndrome. Treatment with the Potassium and Magnesium Salts of Aspartic Acid." 4:98.

Frithiof, et al. 1980. "The Relationship Between Marginal Bone Loss and Serum Zinc Levels." *ACTA Med Scand* 27:67.

Fuchs, N. K. July 1985. "Magnesium: The Key to Calcium Absorption." *Let's Live.*

Gallagher, J. C., and B. L. Riggs. 1978. "Current Concepts in Nutrition: Nutrition and Bone Disease." *New England Journal of Medicine* 298:193.

Gallagher, J. C., et al. 1979. "Intestinal Calcium Absorption and Serum Vitamin D Metabolites in Normal Subjects and Osteoporotic Patients." *Journal of Clinical Investigation* 64:729.

Galland, L. 1986. "Increased Requirements for Essential Fatty Acids in Atopic Individuals: A Review with Clinical Descriptions." *Journal of American College of Nutrition* 5(2):213.

Gambrell, R. D., et al. 1983. "Decreased Incidence of Breast Cancer in Postmenopausal Women: Estrogen-Progestogen." *Journal of Obstetrics & Gynecology* 62:435.

Gambrell, R. D., and R. B. Greenblatt. 1979. "The Menopause: Indications for Estrogen Therapy." *Year Book Medical Publisher*.

Gambrell, R. D. 1987. "Use of Progestogen Therapy." *American Journal of Obstetrics and Gynecology* 156:1304.

Glen, I., et al. February 1987. "The Role of Essential Fatty Acids in Alcohol Dependence and Tissue Damage." *Alcoholism* (NY) 11(1):37.

Goodnight, S. H. 1989. "The Effects of Omega-3 Fatty Acids on Thrombosis and Atherogenesis." *Hematologic Pathology* 3(1):1.

Greenblatt, R. B., and J. C. Emperaire. 1970. "Changing Concepts in the Management of the Menopause." *Medical Times* 98:153.

Greenblatt, R. B. 1963. "Estrogen Therapy for Postmenopausal Females." *New England Journal of Medicine* 272:305.

Greenblatt, R. B., et al. 1982. "Fibrocystic Breast Disease: Current Status of Diagnosis and Treatment." *Postgraduate Medicine* 71:159.

Hain, A. M., and J. C. B. Sym. 1943. "The Control of Menopausal Flushes by Vitamin E." *British Medicine Journal* 7:9.

Hanset, A. E., et al. 1947. "Eczema and Essential Fatty Acids." *American Journal of Diseases of Children* 73:1.

Harris, C. 1957. "The Vicious Cycle of Anemia and Menorrhagia." *Canadian Medical Association Journal* 77:98.

Harrison, M., et al. 1961. "Calcium Metabolism in Osteoporosis." *Lancet* 5:1015.

Haspels, et al. 1978. "Disturbance of Tryptophan Metabolism and its Correction During Oestrogen Treatment in Postmenopausal Women." *Maturitas* 1:15.

Haspels, et al. 1975. "Estrogens and Vitamin B6." Front. Hormone Res., 3:199.

Hayakawa, R., et al. 1981. "Effects of Combination Treatment with Vitamin E and C on Chloasma Pigmented Contact Dermatitis. A Double Blind Control Clinical Trial." *ACTA Vitaminol Enzymol* 3n.s.(1):31.

Hernell, Q., et al. 1982. "Suspected Faulty Essential Fatty Acid Metabolism in Sjogren-Larrson Syndrome." *Pediatric Research* 16:45.

Hoeg, J. M., et al. 1984. "Normalization of Plasma Lipoprotein Concentrations in Patients with Type II Hyperlipoprotenemia by Combined Use of Neomycin and Niacin." *Circulation* 7:1004.

Hollander, D., and A. Tarmawski. March 1986. "Dietary Essential Fatty Acids and the Decline in Peptic Ulcer Disease." *Gut* 22(3):239.

Horrobin, D. F. September 1980. "A Biochemical Basis for Alcoholism and Alcohol-Induced Damage Including the Fetal Alcohol Syndrome and Cirrhosis: Interference with Essential Fatty Acid and Prostaglandin Metabolism." *Medical Hypotheses* 6(9):929.

Horrobin, D. F. 1980. "Essential Fatty Acid and Prostaglandin Metabolism in Sjögren's Syndrome, Systemic Sclerosis and Rheumatoid Arthritis." *Scandinavian Journal of Rheumatology Supplement* 61:242.

Horrobin, D. F. April 1989. "Essential Fatty Acids and the Complications of Diabetes Mellitus." *Wien Klin Wochenschr* 101(8):289.

Horrobin, D. F. 1987. "Essential Fatty Acids in Clinical Dermatology." *Journal of the American Academy of Dermatology* 20(6):1045.

Horrobin, D. F. October–December 1980. "The Regulation of Prostaglandin Biosynthesis by the Manipulation of Essential Fatty Acid Metabolism." *Revue of Pure and Applied Pharmacologic Science* 4(4):339.

Horrobin, D. F. July 1983. "The Role of Essential Fatty Acids and Prostaglandins in the Premenstrual Syndrome." *Journal of Reproductive Medicine* 28(7):465.

Horsman, A., et al. 1977. "Prospective Trial of Oestrogen and Calcium in Postmenopausal Women." *British Medical Journal* 2:789.

Hyams, M. N., and P. D. Gallaher. 1950. "Vitamin A Therapy in the Treatment of Vulvar Leucoplakia." *American Journal of Obstetrics and Gynecology* 59:1346.

Jowsey, J. 1976. "Osteoporosis: Its Nature and the Role of Diet." *Postgraduate Medicine* 60(2):75.

Kaye, W. H., et al. 1982. "Modest Facilitation of Memory in Dementia with Combined Lecithin and Anticholinesterase Treatment." *Biological Psychiatry* 17:275.

Keddie, F. 1948. "Use of Vitamin A in the Treatment of Cutaneous Diseases." *Archives of Dermatology and Syphilology* 58:64.

Klauder, J. V. 1960. "Treatment of Dermatoses with Local Injections of Vitamin A." *AMA Archives of Dermatology* 81:131.

Krouse, T. B., et al. 1979. "Age-Related Changes Resembling Fibrocystic Disease in Iodine-Blocked Rat Breasts." *Archives of Pathology and Laboratory Medicine* 103:631.

Kruse, C. A. 1961. "Treatment of Fatigue with Aspartic Acid Salts." *Northwest Medicine* 6:597.

Larsson, B., et al. July 1989. "Evening Primrose Oil in the Treatment of Premenstrual Syndrome. A Pilot Study." *Current Therapeutic Research* 46:58.

Lee, C. J., et al. 1981. "Effects of Supplementation of the Diets with Calcium and Calcium Rich Food on Bone Density of Elderly Females with Osteoporosis." *American Journal of Clinical Nutrition* 34:819.

Lehman, J. 1973. "Tryptophan Malabsorption in Levodopa-Treated Parkinsonian Patients." *ACTA Med Scand* 194:181.

Lindquist, O. 1982. "Influence of the Menopause on Ischemic Heart Disease and its Risk Factors and on Bone Mineral Content." *ACTA Obstetrica et Gynecologica Scandinavica* 110:7.

Lithgow, P. M., and W. M. Politzer. 1977. "Vitamin A in the Treatment of Menorrhagia." *South African Medical Journal* 51:191.

London, R. F., et al. 1981. "Endocrine Parameters in Alpha-Tocopheryl Therapy of Patients with Mammary Dysplasia." *Cancer Research* 41:3811.

London, R. S., et al. 1976. "Mammary Dysplasia: Clinical Response and Urinary Excretion of 11-Deoxy-17-Ketosteroids and Pregnanediol Following Alpha-Tocopherol Therapy." *Breast* 4:19.

Lutz, J. 1984. "Calcium Balance and Acid Base Status of Women as Affected by Increased Protein Intake and by Sodium Bicarbonate Ingestion." *American Journal of Clinical Nutrition* 39:20.

Machtey, I., and L. Ouaknine. 1978. "Tocopherol in Osteoarthritis: A Controlled Pilot Study." *Journal of the American Geriatrics Society* 26:328.

Malkiel-Shapiro, B. 1958. "Further Observations on Parenteral Magnesium Sulfate Therapy in Coronary Heart Disease." *South African Medical Journal* 12:1211.

Malkiel-Shapiro, B., et al. 1956. "Parenteral Magnesium Sulphate Therapy." *Medical Proceedings* 9:455.

Manku, M. S., et al. 1979. "Prolactin and zinc effects on rat vascular reactivity: Possible relationship to dihomogammalinolenic acid and to prostaglandin synthesis." *Endocrinology* 104:774.

Mansel, R. E., et al. "The Use of Evening Primrose Oil in Mastalgia." *Clinical Uses of Essential Fatty Acids*. Edited by D. F. Horrobin. Montreal, Eden Press, 1983.

Marcus, R. 1982. "The Relationship of Dietary Calcium to Maintenance of Skeletal Integrity of Man: An Interface of Endocrinology and Nutrition." *Metabolism* 31:93.

Marshall, D. H., and B. E. C. Nordin. 1977. "The Effects of 1a-Hydroxyvitamin D3 with and without Oestrogens on Calcium Balance in Postmenopausal Women." *Clinical Endocrinology* 7:1595.

Marshall, D. K., et al. 1977. "The Prevention and Managment of Post-Menopausal Osteoporosis." ACTA Obstet Gynecol Second Suppl 65:49.

Mattill, H. A. 1938. "Vitamin E." *Journal of the American Medical Association* 110:1831.

McLaren, H. C. 1949. "Vitamin E in the Menopause." *British Medical Journal* 12:1378.

McNair, P., et al. 1978. "Hypomagnesemia, a Risk Factor in Diabetic Neuropathy." *Diabetes* 27:1075.

Medina, D., and F. Shepherd. 1980. "Selenium-Mediated Inhibition of Mouse Mammary Tumorigenesis." *Cancer Letters* 5:241.

Nachtigall, L. E. 1987. "Cardiovascular Disease and Hypertension in Older Women." *Obstetrics and Gynecology Clinics of North America* 14:89.

Neuringer, M., and W. E. Connor. September 1986. "Omega-3 Fatty Acids in the Brain and Retina: Evidence for Their Essentiality." *Nutrition Revue* 44(9):285.

Nicholson, J. P., and C. M. Resnick. 1984. "Outpatient Therapy of Essential Hypertension with Dietary Calcium Supplementation." *Journal of the American College of Cardiology* 2:616.

Nordin, B. E. G. 1971. "Clinical Significance and Pathogenesis of Osteoporosis." *British Medical Journal* 1:571.

Pearse, H. A., and J. D. Trisler. 1957. "A Rational Approach to the Treatment of Habitual Abortion and Menometorrhagia." *Clinical Medicine* 9:1081.

Pope, G. S., et al. 1953. "Isolation of an Oestrogenic Isoflavone (Biochanin A) from Red Clover." *Chemistry and Industry* 10:1042.

Preuter, G. W. 1961. "A Treatment for Excessive Uterine Bleeding." *Applied Therapeutics* 5:351.

Ramaswamy, P. G., and R. Natarajan. 1984. "Vitamin B6 Status on Patients with Cancer of the Uterine Cervix." *Nutrition and Cancer* 6:176.

Renaud, S., and L. McGregor. 1980. "Essential Fatty Acids and the Platelet Membrane in Relation to Aggregation." *Annals de la Nutrition de l'Alimentation* 34(2):265.

Riggs, L., et al. 1987. "Treatment of Primary Osteoporosis with Fluoride and Calcium: Clinical Tolerance and Fracture Occurrence." *Journal of the American Medical Association* 243:446.

Romney, S. L., et al. 1981. "Retinoids and the Prevention of Cervical Dysplasia." *American Journal of Obstetrics and Gynecology* 141:890.

Rude, R. K., et al. 1985. "Low Serum Concentrations of 1,25-Dihydroxyvitamin D in Human Magnesium Deficiency." *Journal of Clinical Endocrinology and Metabolism* 61:933.

Salaices, M., et al. 1983. "Effects of Verapamil and Manganese on the Vasoconstriction Responses to Noradrenaline, Serotonin and Potassium in Human and Goat Cerebral Arteries." *Biochemical Pharmacology* 32:2711.

Salway, J. G., et al. 1978. "Effect of MyoInositol in Peripheral Nerve Function in Diabetes." *Lancet* 12:1282.

Schrauzer, G. N., and D. Ishmael. 1974. "Effect of Selenium and Arsenic on the Genesis of Spontaneous Mammary Tumors in Inbred C3H Mice." *Annals of Clinical and Laboratory Science* 4:441.

Schrauzer, G. N. 1976. "Selenium and Cancer: A Review." *Bioinorganic Chemistry* 5:275.

Schrauzer, G. N., et al. 1985. "Selenium in the Blood of Japanese and American Women with and without Breast Cancer and Fibrocystic Disease." *Japanese Journal of Cancer Research* 76:374.

Seelig, M. S. 1964. "The Requirements of Magnesium by the Normal Adult." *American Journal of Clinical Nutrition* 14:342.

Shansky, A. 1981. "Vitamin B3 in the Alleviation of Hypoglycemia." *D and Cl* 10:68.

Shute, E. V., et al. 1948. "The Influence of Vitamin E on Vascular Disease." *Surgery, Gynecology and Obstetrics* 86:1.

Shute, E. V. 1937. "Notes on the Menopause." *Canadian Medical Association Journal* 10:350.

Simpson, L. O. April 1988. "The Etiopathogenesis of Premenstrual Syndrome as a Consequence of Altered Blood Rheology: A New Hypothesis (Evening Primrose Oil, Fish Oils)." *Medical Hypotheses* 25(4):189.

Singer, E. 1936. "Effects of Vitamin E Deficiency on the Thyroid Gland of the Rat." *Journal of Physiology* 87:287.

Skrabel, F., et al. 1981. "Low Sodium/High Potassium Diet for Prevention of Hypertension: Probable Mechanisms of Action." *Lancet* 10:895.

Smith, C. J. 1964. "Non-Hormonal Control of Vaso-Motor Flushing in Menopausal Patients." *Chicago Medicine* 67:193.

Smythies, J. R., and J. R. Halsey. 1984. "Treatment of Parkinson's Disease with L-Methionine." *Southern Medical Journal* 77:1577.

Solomon, D., et al. 1972. "Relationship Between Vitamin E and Urinary Excretion of Ketosteroid Fractions in Cystic Mastitis." *Annals of New York Academy of Sciences* 2:3:103.

Stone, K. J., et al. 1979. "The Metabolism of Dihomogammalineolenic Acid in Man." *Lipids* 14:174.

Taylor, F. A. 1956. "Habitual Abortion: Therapeutic Evaluation of Citrus Bioflavonoids." *Western Journal of Surgery, Obstetrics and Gynecology* 5:280.

Taymor, M. L., et al. 1964. "The Etiological Role of Chronic Iron Deficiency in Production of Menorrhagia." *Journal of the American Medical Association* 187:323.

Taymor, M. L., et al. 1960. "Menorrhagia Due to Chronic Iron Deficiency." *Obstetrics and Gynecology* 16:571.

Tee Khaw K, Thom S. 1962. "Randomized Double-Blind Cross-Over Trial of Potassium on Blood-Pressure in Normal Subjects." *Lancet* 9:1127.

Vles, R. O. 1980. "Essential Fatty Acids in Cardiovascular Physiopathology." *Annales de la Nutrition et de l'Alimentation* 34(2):255.

Wasserthiel-Smoller, S., et al. 1981. "Dietary Vitamin C and Uterine Cervical Dysplasia." *American Journal of Epidemiology* 114:714.

Watson, E. M. 1936. "Clinical Experiences with Wheat Germ Oil (Vitamin E)." *Canadian Medical Association Journal* 2:134.

Wertz, P. W., et al. 1987. "Essential Fatty Acids and Epidermal Integrity." *Archives of Dermatology* 123(10):1381.

Whitacre, F. E., and B. Barrera. 1944. "War Amenorrhea." *Journal of the American Medical Association* 124:399.

Wiley-Rosett, J. A., et al. 1984. "Influence of Vitamin A on Cervical Dysplasia and Carcinoma in situ." *Nutrition and Cancer* 6(1):49.

Wurtman, R. J., et al. 1977. "Lecithin Consumption Raises Serum-Free Choline Levels." *Lancet* 7:68.

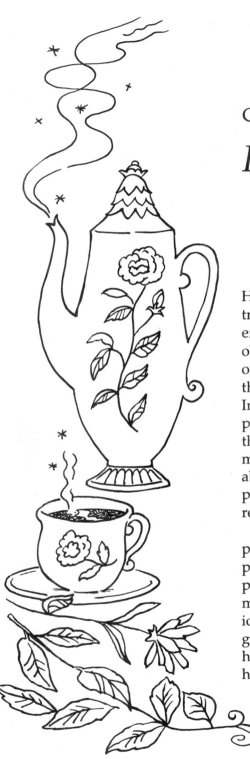

CHAPTER 10

Herbs for Menopause

Herbs were humankind's first medicine and formed the basis of traditional healing practices for thousands of years. Their benficial effects were discovered slowly through trial and error. By careful observation, early cultures learned to recognize the healing effects of medicinal plants for a variety of illnesses and learned to avoid the use of others because of their poisonous or harmful side effects. In modern times many research studies in the fields of botany, pharmacology, and medicine have allowed us to better understand the beneficial effects of many plant substances. Many interesting medical studies have shown that the traditional body of knowledge about herbs was correct in assigning healing properties to many plants. (See the bibliography at the end of this chapter for a list of research studies on herbs.)

Herbs can be a very useful part of your nutritional program to prevent or help balance a variety of symptoms related to menopause. They should be thought of as a form of extended nutrition, providing many nutrients that are necessary for good health in the menopause years. For example, dulse and kelp provide valuable iodine for optimal thyroid function, and red raspberry leaves are a good source of calcium and magnesium. Plants also contain natural hormones and a variety of substances that help to control bleeding, hot flashes, anxiety, insomnia, and other common menopause symptoms. In the following section I will give information on specific herbs that can help relieve menopause symptoms.

Herbs for Your Menopause Symptoms

Heavy irregular menstrual bleeding. Plants that contain bioflavonoids help to strengthen capillaries and prevent heavy, irregular menstrual bleeding (menorrhagia). This is a common bleeding pattern as women approach menopause. Flavonoids are found in a large variety of fruits and flowers and are responsible for their color. Excellent sources are citrus fruits, cherry, grape, and hawthorn berry. According to research studies, they have also been found in red clover and subterranean clover strains in Australia. Many medical studies of citrus bioflavonoids have demonstrated their usefulness in a variety of bleeding problems, besides those related to menopause, such as habitual spontaneous abortion and tuberculosis.

Hot flashes. Many plants are good sources of estrogen, the hormone that helps to control hot flashes. Besides controlling heavy menstrual bleeding, bioflavonoids also have weak estrogenic activity (1/50,000 the strength of estrogen). They are very effective in controlling such common menopause symptoms as hot flashes, anxiety, and irritability. Plants containing bioflavonoids may be particularly useful for women who cannot take supplements because of their concern with the strong side effects of the prescription hormones (increased risk of stroke, cancer, etc.). Other plants sources of estrogen and progesterone used in traditional herbology include dong quai, black cohosh, blue cohosh, unicorn root, false unicorn root, fennel, anise, sarsaparilla, and wild yam root. The hormonal activities of these plants have been studied in a number of interesting research studies.

Plants may also form the basis for the production of medical hormones. Many common plants such as soy beans and yams contain a preformed steroidal nucleus. Estrogen and progesterone can be synthesized from plants in relatively few steps and have allowed sex hormones to become available commercially at a reasonable cost.

Menopause anxiety, irritability, and insomnia. Women with menopause anxiety, irritability, and insomnia have a number of herbal remedies to choose from for relief of their symptoms. Herbs such as passionflower and valerian root have a significant calming and restful effect on the central nervous system. Passionflower has been found to elevate levels of the neurotransmitter serotonin. Serotonin is synthesized from tryptophan, an essential amino acid that has been found in numerous medical studies to initiate sleep and decrease awakening. Valerian root has been used extensively in traditional herbology as a sleep inducer. It is used widely in Europe as an effective treatment for insomnia. Research studies have confirmed both the sedative effect of valerian root and its effectiveness as a means to treat insomnia. For women with menopause insomnia, valerian root can be a real blessing. I have used it with patients for the past fourteen years and noted much symptom relief. Other effective herbal treatments include camomile, hops, catnip, and peppermint teas. I have used all of them in my practice and many pleased patients have commented on their effectiveness.

Menopause fatigue and depression. For women with menopause fatigue and depression, herbs such as oat straw, ginger, cayenne pepper, dandelion root, siberian ginseng (eleutherococcus), and blessed thistle may have a stimulatory effect, improving energy and vitality. Women who use these herbs may note an increased ability to handle stress, as well as improved physical and mental capabilities. Some of the salutory effects may be due to the high levels of the essential nutrients contained in herbs. For example, dandelion root contains magnesium, potassium, and vitamin E, while cayenne has high levels of magnesium and bioflavonoids. These are essential nutrients that have been found to help relieve menopause fatigue, depression, and hot flashes in a number of research studies. Siberian ginseng, ginger, and licorice root have been important traditional medicines in China and other countries for thousands of years. They have been reputed to increase longevity and decrease fatigue and weakness. These herbs have been used to boost immunity and to strengthen the cardiovascular system. In modern China, Japan, and other countries there has been much interest in the pharmacological effects of these traditional herbs. Scientific studies are corroborating the important medicinal effects of these plants. Oat straw has been found in research studies to relieve fatigue and weakness, particularly when there is an emotional component.

Menopause urinary tract symptoms. Many herbs appear to have an ability to soothe, relieve irritation and reduce infection in the urinary tract, including goldenseal, uva ursi, blackberry root, and wintergreen. Research studies suggest that the plant coleus forskohlii also decreases urinary tract pain and discomfort. The urinary tract is a particularly vulnerable area in women during the menopause years and beyond because the lack of hormonal support causes the tissues to become more delicate and easily traumatized. Goldenseal contains berberine, an alkaloid with antibiotic activity, while uva ursi contains arbutin, a urinary diuretic and anti-infective agent. Coleus forskohlii contains forskolin, an antispasmodic which can relieve painful urination as well as menstrual cramps and intestinal colic.

Menopause and sexual frigidity. Herbs have also been popular treatments for the relief of sexual frigidity and impotence. Many cultures hold certain plants in high esteem for their aphrodisiac properties. On closer inspection, some of these plants, like spanish fly or nutmeg, have been found to be genitourinary irritants, rather than sexual stimulants. Traditional Indian medicine considers a number of plants such as saffron crocus and priya-darsa to have extraordinary aphrodisiac powers. Yohimbe, a plant aphrodisiac, is the base of several drugs currently prescribed to treat impotence.

Menopause Herbal Formulas

I have used herbs in my medical practice for years as a form of extended nutrition for menopause. They are an effective means of balancing the diet and optimizing the nutritional intake. There are three herbal formulas that I use to provide optimal nutritional support for women suffering from menopause-related complaints. Formula I can be used by women with general menopause complaints such as hot flashes and vaginal dryness due to hormonal deficiency. Formula II is very helpful for women with menopause-related fatigue, debility, and weakness. Formula III can be used by women with menopause-related anxiety, irritability, and insomnia. Formula I is the basic herbal formula for menopausal women. Formulas II and III should also be used if you have the symptoms for which are applicable.

Herbal Formula I can be ordered by mail through the Menopause Self Help Center (see coupon at the back of the book). Formula I is also widely available in health food stores through Schiff Products.

Herbal Formula I:	Blue Cohosh
	False Unicorn Root
	Fennel
	Anise
	Blessed Thistle
Herbal Formula II:	Ginger
	Cayenne Pepper
	Siberian Ginseng
	(eleutherococcus)
Herbal Formula III:	Valerian root
	Catnip
	Camomile
	Hops
	Red raspberry leaf

The herbs should be used in small amounts and taken with your meals either in capsule form or in a tea. If you prefer to make a tea, simply empty the capsule into a cup of boiling water and let it steep for a few minutes. Do not drink more than one or two cups of the tea per day.

All foods have the potential for causing distress in some people, and herbs are no exception. They should be discontinued immediately if you notice nausea, vomiting, or diarrhea upon using. These are the most common symptoms of intolerance. The herbs in my formulas are all recommended as being safe for human consumption, but some women seem to have a specific intolerance for various foods, including herbs. If you notice any symptoms that make you uncomfortable after using the herbs, discontinue them immediately.

Herbs for Menopause and Female Health Problems

Symptoms	Herbal Treatments
Menorrhagia	Shepherd's purse
	Hawthorn berry
	Cherry
	Grape skin
	Bilberry
	Red clover
Menopause hot flashes, Vasomotor symptoms	Dong quai
	Black cohosh
	Blue cohosh
	Unicorn root
	False unicorn root
	Fennel
	Sarsaparilla
	Red clover
	Wild yam root
Menopause insomnia and anxiety	Valerian root
	Passion flower
	Peppermint
	Catnip
	Camomile
	Hops

Menopause fatigue, tiredness, and depression	Oat straw Ginger Cayenne pepper Dandelion root Siberian ginseng Blessed thistle
Menopause bladder and lower urinary tract symptoms	Coleus forskohlii (pain) Goldenseal (infections) Uva ursi (infections) Blackberry root (infections) Wintergreen
Osteoporosis	Red raspberry leaf Comfrey
Hypothyroidism	Irish moss Kelp Dulse Sarsaparilla
Breast lumps and tenderness	Alfalfa Kelp Poke root poultices

Plants Used as Starting Materials for Commercial Hormone Synthesis

Plant Source	Preformed Steroidal Nucleus
Soybean	Stigmasterol
Calabas bean	Stigmasterol
Yeast	Ergosterol
Cereal grains	B-Sitosterol
Yams	Diosgenin
Sisal	Hecogenin

Suggested Reading

Books

Colbin, A. *Food and Healing*. New York: Ballantine Books, 1986.

Hasselbring, B., et al. *The Medical Self-Care Book of Women's Health*. New York: Doubleday, 1987.

Hylton, W. *The Rodale Herb Booke*. Emmaus, Pa.: Rodale Press, 1974.

Lark, Susan, M.D. *Premenstrual Syndrome Self Help Book*. Berkeley, Ca.: Celestial Arts, 1984.

Lewis, W., and M. Elvin-Lewis. *Medical Botany*. New York: Wiley, 1977.

Lust, J. *The Herb Book*. New York: Bantam, 1974.

Murray, M. *The 21st Century Herbal, Volume I*. Bellevue, Wa.: Vita-Line, 1985.

Murray, M. *The 21st Century Herbal, Volume II*. Bellevue, Wa.: Vita-Line, 1985.

Padus, E. *The Woman's Encyclopedia of Health and Natural Healing*. Emmaus, Pa.: Prevention Books, 1981.

Articles

Ammon, H. P. T., and A. B. Muller. 1985. "Forskolin: From Ayurvedic Remedy to a Modern Agent." *Planta Medica* 51:473–7.

Baranov, A. I. 1982. "Medicinal Uses of Ginseng and Related Plants in the Soviet Union: Recent Trends in the Soviet Literature." *Journal of Ethnopharmacology* 6:339–353.

Butler, C. L., and C. H. Costello. 1944. "Pharmacologic Studies. I. Aletris farinosa." *Journal of the American Pharmaceutical Society* 33:177–83.

Costello, C. H., and E. V. Lynn. 1950. "Estrogenic Substances from Plants. I. Glycyrrhiza." *Journal of the American Pharmaceutical Society*. 39:177–80.

Chang, J., et al. 1984. "Effect of Forskolin on Prostanglanding Synthesis by Mouse Resident Peritoneal Macrophages." *European Journal of Pharmacology* 103:303–12.

Chen, E. W., et al. 1955. "Estrogenic Activity of Some Naturally Occurring Isoflavones." *Annals of the New York Academy of Sciences* 61(3):652.

Cohen, J. D., and H. W. Rubin. 1960. "Functional Menorrhagia: Treatment with Bioflavonoids and Vitamin C." *Current Therapeutic Research* 2(11):539.

Dansi, A., et al. 1937. "The estrogenic activity of polymerized anol." *Biochimica e Terapia Sperimentale* 24:282–284.

Dodds, E. C., and W. Lawson. 1937. "Estrogenic Activity of p-hydroxypropenyl-benzene (anol)." *Nature* 139:1069.

Dodds, E. C., and W. Lawson. 1937. "A Simple Oestrogenic Agent with an Activity of the Same Order as that of Oestrone." *Nature* 139:627.

Elghamry, M. I., and I. M. Shihata. 1965. "Biological Activity of Phytoestrogens." *Planta Medica* 13:352–7.

Faber, K. 1958. "The Dandelion—Taraxacum Officinale Weber." *Pharmazie* 13:423–35.

Gibson, M. R. 1978. "Glycyrrhiza in Old and New Perspectives." *Lloydia* 41:348–54.

Gomez, E. T., and C. W. Turner. 1938. "Effect of anol and dihydrotheelin on mammogenic activity of the pituitary gland of rabbits." *Proceedings of the Society for Experimental Biology and Medicine* 39:140–142.

Hahn, F. E., and J. Ciak. 1976. "Berberine." *Antibiotics* 3:577–88.

Harada, M., et al. 1984. "Effect of Japanese angelica root and peony root on uterine contraction in the rabbit in situ." *Journal of Pharmacologic Dynamics* 7:304–11.

Havsteen, B. 1983. "Flavonoids, a Class of Natural Products of High Pharmacological Potency." *Biochemical Pharmacology* 32:1141–8.

Kerouac, R., et al. 1984. "Forskolin Inhibits Histamine Release by Neurotension in the Rat Perfused Hind Limb." *Research Communications Chemical Pathology Pharmacology* 45:310–2.

Kuhnau, J. 1976. "The Flavonoids: A Class of Semi-Essential Food Components: Their Role in Human Nutrition." *World Review of Nutrition and Diet* 24:117–91.

Leathwood, P. D., and F. Chauffard. 1985. "Aqueous Extract of Valerian Reduces Latency to Fall Asleep in Man." *Planta Medica* 54:144–8.

Leathwood, P. D., et al. 1982. "Aqueous Extract of Valerian Root (Valeriani Officinalis L.) Improves Sleep Quality in Man." *Pharmacol. Biochem Behavior* 17:65–71.

Middleton, E. 1984. "The Flavonoids." *Trends in Pharmaceutical Science* 5:335–8.

Pearse, H. A., and J. D. Trisler. 1957. "A Rational Approach to the Treatment of Habitual Abortion and Menometorrhagia." *Clinical Medicine* 9:1081.

Pope, G. S., et al. 1953. "Isolation of an Oestrogenic Isoflavone (Biochanin A) from Red Clover." *Chemistry and Industry* 10:1042.

Potter, D. E., et al. 1985. "Forskolin Suppresses Sympathetic Neuron Function and Causes Ocular Hypotension." *Current Eye Research* 4:87–96.

Preuter, G. W. 1961. "A Treatment for Excessive Uterine Bleeding." *Applied Therapeutics* 5:351.

Puri, H. S. 1971. "Vegetable Aphrodisiacs of India." *Quarterly Journal of Crude Drug Research* 11 (2) 1742–48.

Racz-Kotilla, E., et al. 1974. "The Action of Taraxacum Offinale Extracts on the Body Weight and Diuresis of Laboratory Animals." *Planta Medica* 26:212–7.

Sabir, M., and N. Bhide. 1971. "Study of Some Pharmacologic Actions of Berberine." *Indian Journal of Physical Pharmacology* 15:111–32.

Schumann, E. 1939. "Newer Concepts of Blood Coagulation and Control of Hemorrhage." *American Journal of Obstetrics and Gynecology* 38:1002–7.

Suekawa, M., et al. 1984. "Pharmacological Studies on Ginger. I. Pharmacological actions of Pungent Constituents, (6) gingerol and (6) shogaol." *Journal of Pharmacologic Dynamics* 7:836–48.

Tanaka, S., et al. 1977. "Antinociceptive Substances from the Roots of Angelica Acutiloba." *Arzneim-Forsch* 27:2039–45.

Taylor, F. A. 1956. "Habitual Abortion: Therapeutic Evaluation of Citrus Bioflavonoids." *Western Journal of Surgery, Obstetrics and Gynecology* 5:280.

"Topical and System Contraceptive Agents." *Medical Letters* 1974; 16(9): 37–40.

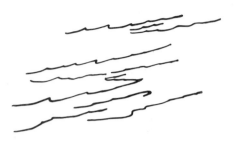

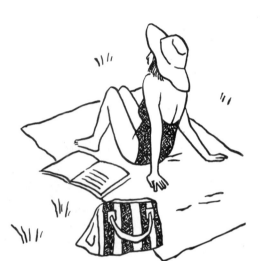

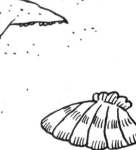

CHAPTER 11

Menopause Stress Reduction

Women in the menopause years may notice that their moods fluctuate more easily. Some women complain that they feel more anxious, irritable, or depressed than usual. They may react with more anger and irritation than usual to problems with their job and family. While by no means universal (some women go through menopause easily with no mood changes at all), it is important to look at both the causes and possible solutions for this problem.

The causes of the mood swings are complex in most women and can be due to physical changes, social and cultural factors, or, more commonly, a combination of both. Some women are very sensitive to the rapid drop in their estrogen and progesterone levels that occur with menopause. They may feel like they are on an emotional roller-coaster as their hormones drop and readjust to a new, lower level.

Another cause of emotional upsets during the menopause period is hypersensitivity of the autonomic nervous system. The autonomic nervous system regulates the bodily functions that we are usually unaware of like pulse rate, respiration, muscle tension, glandular function, and circulation of the blood. The autonomic nervous system is divided into two parts that oppose and complement each other called the sympathetic and parasympathetic nervous systems. For example, if excitement speeds up the heart rate too much, it is the parasympathetic nervous system's job to act as a control circuit and slow it down. If the heart slows down too much, then it is the sympathetic nervous system's job to speed it up. They control the upper and lower limits of your physiology.

Major lifestyle stress that occurs during the mid-life period may cause an overreaction of the sympathetic system. An easily triggered sympathetic nervous system causes your muscles to tense, your blood vessels to constrict, and your heart and pulse rate to speed up so you can react to an emergency. If you have an especially stressful life your sympathetic nervous systems may always be in a state of readiness to react to a crisis. This puts you in a constant state of tension, sometimes known as "fight or flight." You tend to react to small stresses the same way you react to real emergencies. The energy that accumulates in the body to meet this "emergency" must then be discharged, and it is. You may become upset and angry and your system will come into balance once again.

For other women, the social and cultural factors occurring before, during, and after menopause may be quite stressful. Menopause can be a time when children leave home and move away, major career changes are made, and marriage ends in divorce or starts anew. Of course, these major life changes can occur at other times besides the "mid-life crisis," but the combination of hormonal and biochemical changes plus lifestyle changes can be quite difficult to handle.

Since many of these changes, such as the decrease in hormones at menopause, children growing up, or career changes, are unavoidable, it is important to have self-help techniques available that can calm your moods and induce a peaceful and relaxed state of mind. This can be easily achieved through a variety of methods—exercise, meditation, herbal teas, and proper diet and nutritional supplementation. There are many ways for us to alter our own body chemistry toward a healthful balance that feels good. Unfortunately, many women bring their emotional upsets to a doctor's office or do nothing at all, feeling victimized and helpless. Menopausal women who seek help from their doctors for their emotional symptoms may be given strong and potent medications to alter their moods. Often the side effects are worse than the benefits of the medication. Anti-depressants and tranquilizers merely mask the symptoms and never address the causes of the upsets. Strong medication may occasionally be necessary for serious emotional problems, but many women are overmedicated when proper self help techniques can help relieve their symptoms effectively.

Many of my patients have asked me about techniques for coping better with stress. Over the years, I have worked out a strategy that seems to work. I send some women for counseling or psychotherapy, but the majority are looking for practical ways to manage stress on their own. They want to take responsibility for learning to handle their own problems—looking at their methods of dealing with stress, learning techniques to improve their habits and then practicing these techniques on a regular basis. For most women I find that self help techniques are the most effective of all.

Managing Stress

I have found that stress can be managed in four ways:

- Going to a qualified professional for counseling
- Restructuring your environment to make it less stressful
- Learning relaxation and stress-reduction techniques
- Low-stress diet and exercise (discussed elsewhere in the book)

Counseling Services and Support Groups

Look in your city for women's clinics that offer professional counseling services for mid-life women. Many support groups exist that offer peer group support for women in the menopause years. If you are not sure where to find these resources, there is a list at the back of this book that gives the names of national self help groups and newsletters for mid-life women. They are often wonderful sources of information and can direct you to groups in your area.

Restructuring your Environment

If your life seems too complicated because of the stress factors in your life, it may be time to look at your surroundings. Have you created a lifestyle that nurtures you and gives you pleasure? After all, enjoyment of life should be a major goal. Just "getting through the day" is not enough; it's appreciating life's small pleasures and setting up a lovely and loving environment that brings joy to each day. If you go through your day like a robot, simply doing your tasks and enduring discomfort, it's time now to stop and ask yourself what you can do to improve your life.

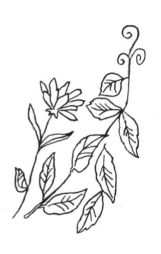

Physical Environment. Have you made your work and home attractive with pictures, plants, or personal accessories? Surrounding yourself with soothing colors and soft music helps you deal with stress. Environmental tapes of ocean sounds, rain falls, or birds chirping can be very relaxing, as can classical music.

Job. Menopause can be a time of career reevaluation. If you dislike your job, try to find another. You might want to take night courses or weekend seminars to prepare yourself for a different field or job level. Even if you can only do this slowly, it will give you something positive to focus on and you'll be learning something that you enjoy. Discuss problems on the job with your boss to see if you can make it a more enjoyable experience.

Work more slowly during the times of day when you begin to drag. Pace yourself, knowing when you tend to experience fatigue. Upgrade your energy during this time by closing your office door or, if you work at home, try going into your bedroom to listen to a relaxation tape, do deep breathing, or meditate. (The specific techniques given in the next section take only a few minutes and can increase your energy tremendously.)

Home. Make your home a nurturing and pleasant place to be. Some homemakers adjust to the empty nest syndrome by getting pets or forming new bonds with women's support groups and

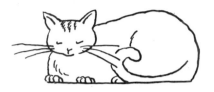

friends. The menopause years are an excellent time to reevaluate and improve your intimate relationships. Do you and your spouse touch and hug one another enough? Do you express your love and appreciation for one another? This can be a time of renewed joy and intimacy in your relationship.

Our intimate relationships can be the most difficult area of all to work on because our relations with our spouses, our children, and ourselves are based almost entirely on our upbringing. We tend to internalize the behavior and beliefs of our own families. We receive these messages very early in life and they are as much a part of us as our arms and legs. A real conflict occurs when what we would like to have as an adult differs from what we have been taught to have. You may want a satisfying sexual relationship, but if your parents didn't have one or taught you that it was to be feared, you may set up your environment so that it doesn't occur. You may fight with your spouse to avoid intimacy, or you may pick a spouse who is not interested in sex. These are just a few of the hundreds of ways that people unconsciously set themselves up for frustration and stress.

If you are extremely uncomfortable with the personal life that you've constructed for yourself, you may need to work with a counselor. On a day-to-day level, however, there are certainly things that you can do to improve your life. Reading psychology books and inspirational texts can help, as can listening to tapes and repeating affirmations to replace the negative parental messages that you learned as a child. Your belief system can slowly be programmed toward what will make you happy.

Techniques for Relaxation

The self help techniques for stress reduction are the most important part of this chapter. If you have symptoms of menopause emotional upset, use these techniques on a daily basis. They can really help you feel better. I recommend breaking up the tasks of the day with these exercises; you will feel much more relaxed.

The tendency to feel rushed and tense is built in to our culture. We in the West tend to be very goal-oriented. We hurry through the day trying to complete tasks as quickly as possible, and then go on to the next ones. There is a continual sense of urgency—"I've got to get it done"—without much regard for how we get there. This tends to speed up the autonomic nervous system responses that lead to stress and tension and which can worsen menopause symptoms. With the use of relaxation techniques, tasks get done in the same amount of time and the journey is much more enjoyable.

I have made a point of working in a relaxed and unhurried way while I write this book. I have found that when I work in a rushed manner, I become more nervous and tired by the end of the day. My back muscles feel sore from bending over the computer. If I work in a leisurely way, I get out of my chair every hour or two and take a break. I stretch my cramped muscles, do some deep-breathing exercises, and clear out my mind. The surprise is that I get more work done the second way— and feel much more relaxed and energetic at the end of the workday.

I have been teaching these relaxation methods to patients for many years. We go over the exercises at my office, or they learn them on their own using the books and tapes that I suggest. Almost without exception the patients come back very enthusiastic about the results: they say the exercises calm their minds and bodies, they feel happier and more positive about their lives, and they note improvements in their physical health. A calm mind seems to calm the body: the autonomic nervous system slows down and the body chemistry normalizes.

Here are some simple exercises that I have found to be very helpful for women with menopause.

First step: Find a comfortable position. For many women, this means lying on their backs. You may also do the exercises sitting up. Try to keep your spine as straight as possible. Your arms and legs should be uncrossed. It is important that your clothes be loose and comfortable.

Second step: Focus your attention upon the exercises so that distracting thoughts do not interfere with your concentration. Close your eyes and take a few deep breaths, in and out. This will help to quiet your mind and remove your thoughts from the problems and tasks of the day.

Exercise 1: Deep Abdominal Breathing

Deep, slow abdominal breathing is very important for your health and vitality. It brings adequate oxygen, the fuel for metabolic activity, to all the tissues of your body. Rapid, shallow breathing decreases our oxygen supply and keeps us devitalized. Deep breathing helps to relax the entire body and strengthens the muscles in the chest and abdomen.

- Lie flat on your back with your knees pulled up. Keep your feet slightly apart. Try to breathe in and out through your nose.

- Inhale deeply. As you breathe in, allow your stomach to relax so that the air flows into your abdomen. Your stomach should balloon out as you breathe in. Visualize your lungs filling up with air so that your chest swells out.

- Imagine that the air you breathe is filling your body with energy.

- Exhale deeply. As you breathe out, let your stomach and chest collapse. Imagine the air being pushed out, first from your abdomen and then from your lungs.

Exercise 2: Color Breathing

Color breathing has traditionally been used to heal the body, calm the nerves, and strengthen the body's energy field. Ancient Indian and oriental spiritual traditions described the body's energy field in detail as far back as 3,000 B.C. Intuitives in our culture are able to describe the energy field as lights or colors that emanate from the body. Different parts of the body appear to emanate different colors: the legs emanate red, the pelvis and intestines orange, the solar plexus yellow, the heart green, the throat blue, the eyes and pituitary violet, and the top of the head white. Each color is thought to give energy and strength to the body part to which it corresponds.

When you are calm and relaxed, the human energy field looks radiant, harmonious, and full of color. It has the soft rounded shape of an Easter egg. Emotional imbalances such as anxiety, irritability, insomnia, and depression that can occur during the menopause time can upset the energy field, creating disturbances in its colors, intensity, and shape. Color breathing is a powerful technique to calm the mind and the body as well as to balance the energy field.

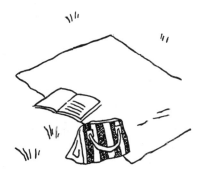

- Sit or lie in a comfortable position. Imagine that the earth beneath you is filled with the color red. This color goes several hundred feet below you into the earth. Visualize your body drawing this red color in. As you inhale slowly, breathe the red into your body. See it come up through your feet, legs, abdomen, trunk, arms, neck, and head. See it fill the air around you. Exhale the red slowly out your lungs. Repeat this process slowly five times.

- Now see the color orange filling the earth beneath you. As you inhale, move it from the earth up into your body, starting with your feet. Fill the air around you with orange. As you exhale, breathe orange out of your lungs. Do this five times. Repeat the exercise with the colors yellow, green, blue, violet, and white.

Exercise 3: Discovering Muscle Tension

Many women have muscles that are chronically tight and tense. Tense muscles get inadequate blood flow and oxygen, and accumulate an excess of lactic acid. We often carry these habitual patterns of tension for years and feel as if parts of our body are locked in a vise. Because the way our body feels can have a profound effect on our moods, women with chronically tight muscles tend to be more "uptight" and irritable. Movement is the most effective antidote to this tension because it improves circulation and helps to break up habitual patterns of muscle holding and contracting. Unfortunately, the problem is accentuated in many women in the menopause years, as they become less active with age and lead more sedentary lives, instead of engaging in sports or other physical activities. They sit instead of standing and drive when they could walk. When our muscles are loose, limber, and have a full range of movement we tend to feel lighter and more relaxed. Anxiety disappears and we are filled instead with peace and calm. The next two exercises will help you to get in touch with your own muscle tension and will aid you in releasing the chronic blocks and holding patterns that can adversely affect your mood.

- Lie in a comfortable position. Allow your right arm to rest limply, palm down, on the surface next to you.

- Now raise just the hand, not the entire arm, and hold it there for 15 seconds. How does the top of your forearm feel? Does it feel tight and tense?

- Now let your arm drop down and relax. The arm muscles will relax too. They should feel comfortable again.

- Now raise your right foot off the floor, pointing your toes straight up. How does your leg feel? Does it feel tight and tense?

- Now let your foot drop down and relax. You will feel the muscles in your legs relax too.

- As you lie there, notice any other parts of your body that carry tension. They will feel tight and a little sore. You may notice a constant dull aching. Tense muscles block blood flow and cut off the supply of nutrients to the tissues. The muscle is poorly oxygenated and in response it produces lactic acid. Go to the next exercise for a muscle relaxation technique.

Exercise 4: Progressive Muscle Relaxation

- Lie in a comfortable position. Allow your arms to rest limply, palms down on the surface next to you. Practice your deep abdominal breathing as you do this exercise.

- Clench your hands into fists and hold them tightly for fifteen seconds. As you do this, relax the rest of your body. Then let your hands relax.

- Now tense and relax the following parts of your body in this order: your face, shoulders, back, stomach, pelvis, legs, feet,

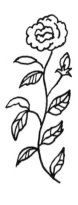

and toes. Hold each part tensed for fifteen seconds and then relax your body for thirty seconds before going on to the next part.

• Visualize the tense part contracting, becoming tighter and tighter. On relaxing, see the energy flowing into the entire body like a gentle wave, making all the muscles soft and pliable.

• Finish the exercise by shaking your hands and imagining the remaining tension flowing out your fingertips.

This is a particularly useful exercise to do when you feel tension building up during the day. It helps to discharge stress in a beneficial way.

Exercise 5: Meditation

• Lie or sit in a very comfortable position.

• Close your eyes and breathe deeply. Let your breathing be slow and relaxed.

• Focus all of your attention on your breathing. Notice the movement of your chest and abdomen in and out.

• Block out all other thoughts, feelings, and sensations. If you feel your attention wandering, bring it back to your breathing.

• Count to one as you inhale, two as you exhale, three as you inhale, four as you exhale, until you reach twenty. Repeat this exercise at least five times. For the best results, repeat the sequence for as long as you are able, up to five minutes.

This meditation requires you to sit quietly and engage in a simple and repetitive activity. (This can be very difficult at first.) By emptying your mind you give yourself a rest. The metabolism of your body slows down. The brainwave slows from the fast beta wave that predominates during the normal working day to a slower alpha or theta wave. This slower pattern is what appears during sleep or in the period of deep relaxation just before falling asleep. Meditating gives the mind a vacation from tension and worry. It is useful to do during the menopause time when every little stress can be magnified.

Exercise 6: Affirmations for Menopause

Sit in a comfortable position. Repeat the following affirmations three times. You may find that you have negative feelings about your body and menopause when repeating certain affirmations. These correspond to deeply held beliefs about your body that you would like to change. This exercise is very effective in helping to change negative and unhappy thoughts to positive thoughts of self-love and acceptance. Keep doing this exercise on a regular basis and it will help you to like your own body more as you go through the changes of menopause. You may find that you want to emphasize certain affirmations and delete others. You may also find that writing each affirmation three times is very effective.

- Menopause is a healthy and happy time for me.
- I love my body as it goes through menopause.
- I go through menopause with ease and comfort.
- My body is strong and healthy.
- My body becomes healthier each day.
- My hormones are perfectly balanced and regulated.
- My body chemistry is healthy and balanced.
- My female system is strong and healthy.
- My female organs are full of health and vitality.
- My breasts are full of health and vitality.
- My thyroid is full of health and vitality.
- My bones and joints are strong and healthy.
- I love my body.
- I feel wonderful as I go through menopause.
- My mood is calm and relaxed.
- I handle stress easily and effortlessly.
- I do my work and activities in a relaxed and comfortable way. They bring me pleasure.

- I take time each day to relax and enjoy myself.
- I practice the relaxation methods that I enjoy.
- I am enjoying my life more and more. My life brings me pleasure.
- I enjoy the company of my family and friends. They give me pleasure.
- I eat a well-balanced and healthful diet.
- I eat the foods that keep my body strong and healthy.
- I enjoy eating the foods that are delicious and full of healthy vitamins and minerals.
- As I get older, I am becoming stronger and healthier.
- I am full of vigor and vitality.
- Each day I practice the self help methods that I enjoy. My life is fun and exciting.

Affirmations are very important because they align your mind with your body. It is not enough during the menopause years and beyond to exercise vigorously and follow an excellent diet; it is also important to like your body and think positive thoughts as you go through the changes related to menopause. This is because your state of health is determined by the interaction between your mind and body, by the thousands of messages you send yourself each day with your thoughts. For example, if you do not like yourself and equate menopause with becoming "unattractive," "decrepit," or "falling apart," you will be constantly criticizing yourself—the way you look, talk, and act. This well be reflected in your body: your countenance will be lackluster and depressed, your face will look unhappy and depressed, and your body will be slumped and rounded. Your looks will perfectly match your beliefs.

You can aggravate your menopause symptoms with negative thoughts because when your body believes it is sick, it behaves accordingly. As you can see, it is very important to cultivate a positive belief system and a positive body image.

This technique of imaging your body the way you want it to be has been used to great benefit for patients with many types of diseases. In his book, *Getting Well Again*, Carl Simonton, a cancer radiation therapist, describes how he used this technique with his patients. He asked them to imagine that they had strong immune systems capable of fighting a small, puny cancer (instead of the other way around). In a substantial number of cases he saw patients with very serious diseases go into remission.

Exercise 7: Visualizations for Menopause

This exercise uses visual pictures to achieve a positive body image. It is a very powerful technique that actually lets you see your body in a healthy and vital state.

- Close your eyes. Begin to breathe deeply. Inhale and let the air out slowly. Feel your body begin to relax.

- Imagine yourself looking in a magic mirror that lets you look inside your body. You can see your hands and face, but you can also look inside at your vital organs.

- Look at your female organs. They are full of energy and vitality. Your ovaries, uterus, and vagina are very healthy. They have an attractive pink color. Nutrients and oxygen flow freely to them and they release their waste products out of the body. Your vagina is moist, pink, and healthy. It is elastic and expandable. You are able to enjoy a healthy and active sex life.

- Look at your breasts. They feel perfectly normal. The tissue is smooth and without lumps or masses. They feel comfortable when you touch them.

- Look at your thyroid. It is the gland that sits across your neck in front. It is a healthy size and texture. It is perfectly regulated and functions normally.

- Look at your bones. They are strong and sturdy. They are full of calcium and other essential nutrients.

- Look at your face. It is smooth and relaxed. There is a smile on your face. You feel in command of yourself. You do not feel anxious, irritable, or depressed. Your mood is wonderful. As you

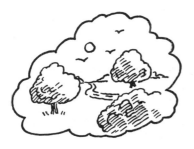

look at yourself in the mirror, you know that you can handle any problems that come along, competently and with great ease.

- Your skin is smooth and moist. Touch your face and hands. You take wonderful care of your skin by using moisturizers, sunscreens, and limiting your sun exposure. Your skin looks lovely.

- Look at your entire body and enjoy the feeling of energy and optimism that is running through you. You are very calm and peaceful.

- Now stop visualizing the scene and go back to deep breathing.

- You open your eyes and feel very good.

- Visualizing this scene should take about forty-five seconds to one minute, perhaps longer if you choose to linger with a particular image. A visualization is successful when it allows you to actually change your feelings about a particular situation.

Your visualization should begin to lay down the mental blueprint for a healthier body and more positive system of beliefs about your health. As you see your body radiating health and looking vital, you actually stimulate the positive chemical changes in your body to help create this condition.

Positive visualization also helps to modify your behavior so that you can create the body pictures you like. You are more likely to choose the foods and nutrients, and to practice the exercises and self-care techniques that benefit the visualizations.

More Stress-Reduction Techniques for Menopause

Hydrotherapy

Warm water has been used for centuries as a way to induce relaxation. Women in Europe would go to spas during the eighteenth and nineteenth centuries to take a series of mineral baths in order to relax and rejuvenate the entire body. Ancient Romans used public baths both as a place to relax and socialize as well as to heal the

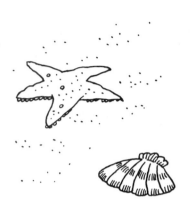

body. You can have your own "spa" at home by adding minerals to a hot bath. Just run a tub of hot water and add one cup of sea salt and one cup of bicarbonate of soda. This is a highly alkaline mixture that should be used only one or two times a month. It is very relaxing and helps to calm menopause anxiety and irritability.

Soak for about twenty minutes. You will probably feel very relaxed and sleepy after this bath. It is best taken just before going to sleep at night. Chances are you will sleep very well. You may wake up feeling refreshed and full of energy the next day.

You can also relax and luxuriate by taking a bubble bath or add scented floral oils to the tub. Turn out the lights, light a candle, and listen to classical music. Many women own hot tubs or have them available through their local health club or YMCA. The combination of heat and water massage from the tub's small powerful jets are very helpful in relaxing tight muscles and reducing tension. It is particularly beneficial for women who suffer from menopause insomnia, since heat appears to induce brainwaves related to deep and restful sleep.

Sound

Music can have a profound and beneficial effect on our moods. Slow, quiet classical music can slow our heart rate, lower our blood pressure, and decrease the amount of stress hormones. It can help to reduce menopause anxiety and induce peaceful sleep for women suffering from insomnia.

Gospel and pop music can elevate our moods and make us want to sing along and dance. It can be a powerful healer to women who note a tendency towards low spirits and depression during the menopause years.

Even tapes and records of nature sounds such as ocean waves and rainfall have the ability to soothe and relax us. I strongly recommend using nonvocal music that suits your mood as an effective means of menopause stress reduction. Play it often at home or in your car as you drive.

Light

Depression and a lowered energy level can make menopause an unhappy time for susceptible women. This is especially true during the winter when days are shorter and less sunlight is available. Medical research has found that moods can be dramatically elevated with the use of full-spectrum fluorescent lights. Light bulbs that approximate daylight are available from Durotest Corporation in North Bergen, New Jersey. I recommend using these lights to extend the daylight hours so that you can approximate summer light. You may find that your moods pick up and you feel much happier.

The full-spectrum light can also help improve calcium absorption by increasing your vitamin D levels. This can be useful in helping to prevent osteoporosis. Much indoor fluorescent light predominates in selected parts of the light spectrum. It is much healthier to be exposed to the whole spectrum, so I would encourage the use of full-spectrum lights for all women. If this is not possible, you can increase your amount of full-spectrum light exposure by opening up your windows and blinds, waking up earlier, and spending more time outdoors.

Putting Your Relaxation Program Together

This chapter has introduced you to many different ways to reset your mind and body to help make the menopause period a pleasurable and relaxed time. Try each exercise at least once. Experiment with them until you find the combination that works for you. Doing all seven will take no longer than twenty to thirty minutes, depending on how much time you wish to spend with each one. Ideally, the exercises should be done on a daily basis for at least a few minutes a day. Over time, they will help you to gain insight into your negative beliefs and change them into positive new ones. Your ability to cope with stress should be tremendously improved.

Suggested Reading

Benson, Robert, and Miriam Klipper. *Relaxation Response*. New York: Avon, 1976.

Brennan, Barbara Ann. *Hands of Light*. New York: Bantam, 1987.

Davis, Martha McKay, and Mathew and Elizabeth Eshelman. *The Relaxation and Stress Reduction Workbook*. Oakland, Ca.: New Harbinger Publications, 1982.

Gawain, Shakti. *Creative Visualization*. San Rafael, Ca.: New World Publishing, 1978.

Gawain, Shakti. *Living in the Light*. Mill Valley, Ca.: Whatever Publishing, 1986.

Kripalu Center for Holistic Health. *The Self-Health Guide*. Lenox, Ma.: Kripalu Publications, 1980.

Loehr, James, and Jeffrey Migdow. *Take a Deep Breath*. New York: Villard Books, 1986.

Miller, Emmett. *Self Imagery*. Berkeley, Ca.: Celestial Arts, 1986.

Ray, Sondra. *I Deserve Love*. Berkeley, Ca.: Celestial Arts, 1976.

Ray, Sondra. *The Only Diet There Is*. Berkeley, Ca.: Celestial Arts, 1981.

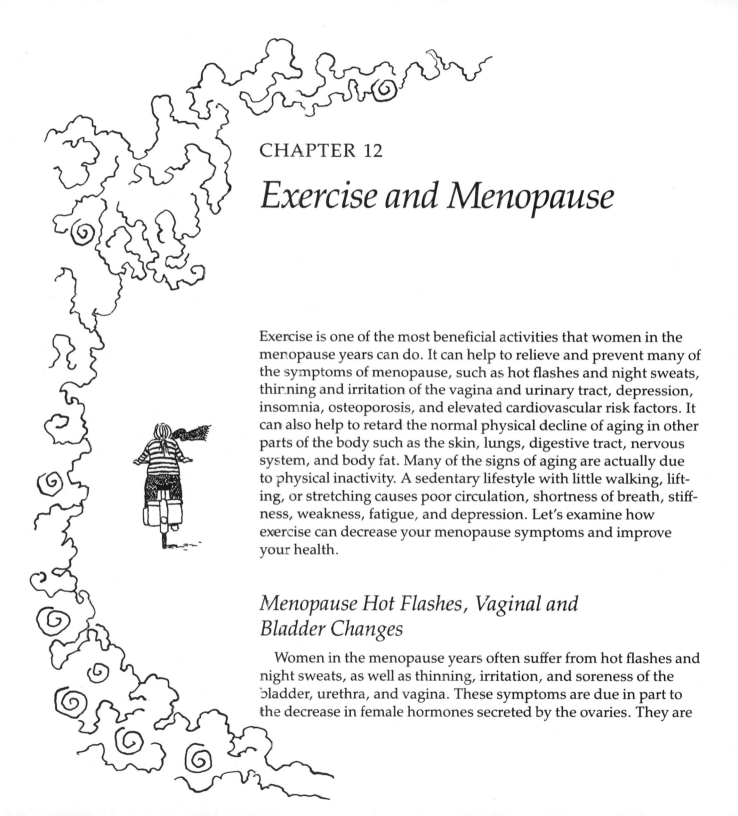

CHAPTER 12

Exercise and Menopause

Exercise is one of the most beneficial activities that women in the menopause years can do. It can help to relieve and prevent many of the symptoms of menopause, such as hot flashes and night sweats, thinning and irritation of the vagina and urinary tract, depression, insomnia, osteoporosis, and elevated cardiovascular risk factors. It can also help to retard the normal physical decline of aging in other parts of the body such as the skin, lungs, digestive tract, nervous system, and body fat. Many of the signs of aging are actually due to physical inactivity. A sedentary lifestyle with little walking, lifting, or stretching causes poor circulation, shortness of breath, stiffness, weakness, fatigue, and depression. Let's examine how exercise can decrease your menopause symptoms and improve your health.

Menopause Hot Flashes, Vaginal and Bladder Changes

Women in the menopause years often suffer from hot flashes and night sweats, as well as thinning, irritation, and soreness of the bladder, urethra, and vagina. These symptoms are due in part to the decrease in female hormones secreted by the ovaries. They are also worsened, however, by poor muscle tone and blood circulation in the pelvic area. This can be remedied by vigorous physical activity such as walking, swimming, tennis, and other sports that cause a vigorous pumping action of the muscles. This brings blood flow, oxygen, and nutrients to the pelvic area and helps to keep the tissues healthy. Regular sexual activity either through intercourse or masturbation can make you feel better. For the same reason, women who remain sexually active show fewer signs of vaginal aging than celibate women. Even loving touch can improve circulation to the pelvic area through massage or gentle stroking of the whole body. This promotes muscle relaxation and improves circulation. This can be done easily by couples, who can give much pleasure to each other through learning simple massage techniques. (A good beginner's manual is *The Book of Massage* by Lidell and Thomas, Fireside Publications.) Single women can exchange massages with friends.

Local exercises of the pelvic area can improve bladder control, vaginal elasticity, and can increase sexual pleasure. Dr. Arnold Kegel developed a set of exercises in the 1940s that all women should practice during the menopause years. The Kegel exercises strengthen the muscles that surround the urethra, vagina, and anus. Women who do these exercises frequently find that they are more aware of their vagina, they report more sensation in the pelvic area, and they find sex more pleasurable. They also notice less leaking of urine when they cough, sneeze, or laugh.

The Kegel exercises are simple and easy to do. They can be done anywhere—sitting, standing, or lying down. They can be performed as follows:

- Draw up the vaginal muscles, hold for three seconds, then relax. Repeat the process five times.
- Then squeeze your vaginal muscles firmly, hold for three seconds, then relax. Repeat the process five times.

Menopause Mood Changes

Exercise can bring significant relief for women who experience menopause anxiety, irritability, or insomnia. Regular exercise promotes a feeling of calmness and relaxation by helping to balance the autonomic nervous system. It also provides an effective way to discharge the overactive "fight and flight" pattern that some women experience around the time of menopause because of the shift in their hormones and body chemistry. Many women note a deep sense of peace and well-being after they exercise. This may be due to an increased output of endorphins, chemicals made by the brain that have a natural opiate effect and are thought to be the reason for the "runner's high" that many marathoners experience. Another benefit of exercise is its promotion of deep, restful sleep—a real plus for women who suffer from menopause insomnia. Exercise may also help women with the opposite problem: menopause depression and fatigue. Some women notice a real decline in their zest and energy level with menopause. They complain that as their hormone levels drop, their joy of living drops also. Vigorous exercise brings blood to the brain, the endocrine glands, and the female reproductive tract. It helps these systems to operate more efficiently and can really help to boost the energy level and relieve depression.

Osteoporosis

Medical studies show that exercise, along with intake of vitamin D and calcium, is an important factor in preventing osteoporosis. When people are physically active, calcium is used efficiently by the body for bone growth and maintenance. Lack of exercise causes people to lose bone as well as muscle mass. This is true even for young people who are confined to bed by an illness. Both upper and lower body must be exercised to maintain thick, strong bones. For women in the menopause years, weight-bearing exercises such as brisk daily walking, dancing, running, and golf are the best ways to maintain bone density in your lower body. To build upper body strength, lifting small two- or three-pound weights can be very helpful. Other activities to build upper body strength include tennis and other regular racket sports, gardening, and even lifting small objects at home like books and cans. The most important thing is to keep moving. Walk instead of sitting down, climb stairs instead of taking the elevator. Avoid prolonged sitting during the day, either at a desk, in front of a TV, or even reading and playing cards. Break up the day with many small "stretch and move sessions"—even five to ten minutes may be very beneficial. This should be in addition to your regular daily exercise.

Heart Disease

Exercise can help to prevent heart disease. Along with a low-fat diet, exercise is routinely prescribed now by doctors for people at high risk of heart disease or recovering from a heart attack. Exercise helps condition the heart and lungs to work more efficiently. A healthy heart is a well-functioning pump. It beats slowly and forcefully, circulating more blood throughout the body with each stroke than does a compromised system. Lungs function more efficiently with exercise, too. They are able to expand more fully and fill with oxygen. Exercise also helps to dilate and expand the network of blood vessels in the body, which allows more blood to reach the muscles and vital organ systems. It also helps to prevent blood clotting and to lower the level of fat in the blood vessels. A healthy heart and lungs mean more endurance and physical energy. You can go through your daily activities more easily, with a sense of vigor and well-being. Exercise that helps to condition the heart and lungs to work more efficiently and utilize oxygen optimally during activity is called *aerobic* exercise.

The best aerobic exercise to tone the heart and lungs is walking three miles a day on a regular basis. This is often the easiest activity for people who do not have athletic facilities near them or lack the time and means to use a gym. Walking is free and is as near as your front door. If possible, find a pleasant walking path in your neighborhood or near a park or school. Other activities that benefit the heart and lungs include swimming, tennis, and dancing. A stationary bicycle is useful in bad weather. Starting a cardiovascular fitness program should be done gradually, particularly if you have not exercised for a while.

I strongly recommend seeing your physician for a cardiovascular risk assessment. This is particularly important if you have a previous history of cardiovascular disease, diabetes mellitus, or high blood pressure. Your physician can identify any potential problems and help you tailor your exercise program.

Weight Control and Appearance

Exercise is important in the menopause years to help keep your weight under control. As our endocrine glands (such as the thyroid and pituitary glands) and our digestive tract age, we tend to slow down and metabolize food less efficiently. We need fewer calories to maintain the same weight. Women who are overweight and inactive complain that they must eat smaller and smaller meals to maintain their weight. Older women who want to maintain their appearance end up in a state of chronic dieting to prevent "middle-age spread." This is not really necessary if an active exercise program is added to a healthful and nutritious diet such as the menopause diet described in chapter 4. Exercise allows you to maintain your weight far more easily because it burns calories and stimulates your metabolism. A regular aerobic program of walking, dancing, swimming, or other activity plus flexibility exercises is a must to control your weight and allow you to look and feel good. A regular exercise program also aids your appearance by helping to preserve attractive body contours by toning your muscles and improving your skin. Exercise increases blood circulation to the skin, which helps to keep the skin pink, soft, and supple. Skin on a woman who doesn't exercise tends to look pallid.

It is important, however, not to try to be too thin with the onset of menopause. Women who are too thin have lower estrogen levels and tend to be at higher risk for such menopause problems as osteoporosis and hot flashes. Aim for a weight level and appearance that is attractive and not extreme . . . neither too thin nor obese. Set your weight and exercise program at a level that feels comfortable, is easy to maintain, and looks good.

Activity Chart

Lower body exercises	• Walking • Jogging • Hiking • Race Walking
Upper body exercises	• Tennis • Racket Sports
Whole body	• Swimming • Dancing • Tennis • Racket sports • Golf (walking only)
Flexibility exercises	• Yoga • T'ai chi • Dancing
Strength building	• Lifting weights

Benefits of Exercise

- Helps to relieve hot flashes, and vaginal and bladder changes of menopause
- Helps to prevent osteoporosis
- Relieves anxiety, irritability, insomnia, and depression
- Conditions heart, lungs, and muscles
- Helps to prevent heart disease
- Helps control weight, improves appearance
- Improves function of vital organs such as digestive tract and nervous system
- Improves strength, stamina, and flexibility
- Increases vigor and energy

Tips for Staying Active

- Increase the amount of time you walk each day.
- Use stairs, not the elevator.

- If you are going a short distance, walk instead of driving.
- Don't always try to park right next to a store or restaurant. Try parking a short distance away.
- Do your Kegel exercise anytime when standing or sitting.
- Plan get-togethers with friends that are based on an activity. For example, take a walk together, or visit a park. Social activities do not need to always be planned around sedentary activities such as meals or playing cards.
- With sedentary activities such as watching television or reading, be sure to take several short breaks to do five minutes of stretching and flexibility exercise.
- Plan a regular exercise program that incorporates aerobic exercise such as walking, bicycling, swimming, or tennis with flexibility exercises.

General Fitness and Flexibility Exercises for Menopause

The following set of exercises will give you a self help program that you can use to promote mobility, flexibility, and relaxation. These gentle exercises are particularly helpful for women during the menopause years because they will help to loosen all the joints in the body and decrease stiffness and soreness.

Doing these exercises on a regular basis will also help improve your vigor and energy level. They can be used as warmups to prepare you for the specific exercises to help correct your menopause symptoms. They should also be used to warm up tense and tight muscles before engaging in sports or athletic events.

I do these exercises as soon as I get out of bed in the morning. They loosen me up and help me start my day right. I find that they even affect my zest and enthusiasm for the tasks of the day.

How to Perform the General Fitness and Flexibility Exercises

1. These exercises should be done the first week or two of your program. Try each warmup exercise at least once, then put

together your own routine. You may find that you want to do all of them on a regular basis, or perhaps only a few. Warm-ups should always precede any sports or athletic events.

2. The exercises should be performed in a relaxed and unhurried manner. Be sure to set aside adequate time—thirty minutes or less—so that you do not feel rushed. Your work area should be quiet, peaceful, and uncluttered.

3. Choose a flat area and work on a mat or a blanket. This will make you more comfortable while you do the exercises.

4. Wear loose, comfortable clothing. It is better that you work without socks to give your feet complete freedom of movement and to prevent slipping.

5. Evacuate your bowels or bladder before you begin the exercises. Wait at least two hours after eating to exercise.

6. Try to practice these movements on a regular basis. A short session every day is best. If that is not possible, then try to practice them every other day.

7. Pay close attention to the initial instructions when beginning an exercise. Look at the placement of the body as shown in the photographs. This is very important, for you are much more likely to have relief of your symptoms if the exercise is practiced properly.

8. Try to visualize the exercise in your mind, then follow with proper placement of the body.

9. Move slowly through the exercise. This will help promote flexibility of the muscles and prevent injury.

10. Always rest for a few minutes after doing the exercises.

General Fitness and Flexibility

Exercise 1: Deep Abdominal Breathing

Proper breathing is essential for deep relaxation, abundant energy, and stress control. This means that you breathe slowly and deeply, filling up your lungs and abdomen. The following exercise will help you to do this.

1. Lie flat on your back with your knees pulled up. Keep your feet slightly apart. Breathe in and out through your nose.

2. Inhale deeply. As you breathe in, allow your stomach to relax so that the air flows into your abdomen. Your stomach should balloon out as you breathe in. Visualize the lowest part of your lungs filling up with air.

3. Imagine that the air you breathe is filling your body with energy.

4. Exhale deeply. As you breathe out, imagine the air being pushed out from the bottom of your lungs to the top, as if a tube of toothpaste were being rolled up.

Exercise 2: Joint Flexibility

Stiffness and soreness in the muscle and joints are common as women age. This is usually due to inactivity, poor habits of posture, stress, chronic patterns of injury, and disease.

The following exercise is designed to remedy these problems by improving the range of motion and flexibility in all the major joints of the body. The gentle stretching of the muscles around the joints will help to reduce tension and stress. These stretches are also thought to open and stimulate the acupuncture meridians based on the work of Motoyama, a distinguished Japanese researcher, as described in his book, *Theories of the Chakras: Bridge to Higher Consciousness*.

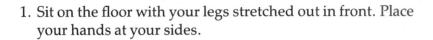

1. Sit on the floor with your legs stretched out in front. Place your hands at your sides.

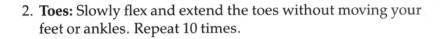

2. **Toes:** Slowly flex and extend the toes without moving your feet or ankles. Repeat 10 times.

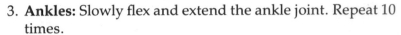

3. **Ankles:** Slowly flex and extend the ankle joint. Repeat 10 times.

    Separate your legs slightly, then rotate your ankles in each direction 10 times. Be sure to keep your heels on the floor.

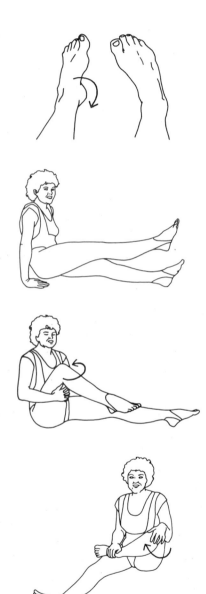

4. **Knees:** Still resting in the sitting position, bend the right leg at the knee, bringing the heel near the right buttock.

    Then lift the right leg off the ground, straightening the right knee. Repeat 10 times. Then do the same exercise with the left leg.

    Hold the thigh near the chest with both hands. Rotate your lower leg in a circular motion about the knee 10 times clockwise and then 10 times counterclockwise. Repeat with the left leg.

5. **Hips:** Bend the left leg so that you can place your left foot on the right thigh. Hold the left knee with the left hand and hold the left ankle with the right hand. Then gently move the left knee up and down with the left hand. Repeat with the right leg.

    While you are sitting in the same position, rotate the left knee clockwise 10 times and then counterclockwise 10 times. This improves the flexibility of the hip joints. Repeat on the right side.

    While sitting, bring the soles of the feet together, bringing the heels close to the body. Using the hands, put the knees to the floor and then let them come up again. Repeat 10 times.

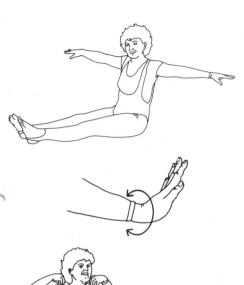

6. **Fingers:** Sit on the floor with your legs stretched out in front. Lift your arms up to shoulder height, keeping them straight. Open the hands wide. Flex the fingers, closing them over the thumbs to make a fist. Repeat 10 times.

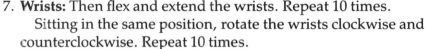

7. **Wrists:** Then flex and extend the wrists. Repeat 10 times.
   Sitting in the same position, rotate the wrists clockwise and counterclockwise. Repeat 10 times.
   Sitting in the same position, hold the hands in extension and move the hand from side to side at the wrist. Repeat 10 times.

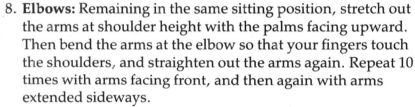

8. **Elbows:** Remaining in the same sitting position, stretch out the arms at shoulder height with the palms facing upward. Then bend the arms at the elbow so that your fingers touch the shoulders, and straighten out the arms again. Repeat 10 times with arms facing front, and then again with arms extended sideways.

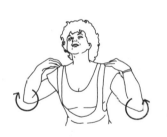

9. **Shoulders:** From the same sitting position, with the arms bent and the fingertips touching the shoulders, make a circular motion with the elbows. Repeat 10 times clockwise and 10 times counterclockwise.

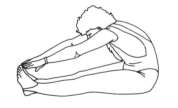

10. **Spine:** Remain sitting down with your legs together straight in front of you. Reach over and touch your legs without bending your knees. Repeat 20 times.

11. **Waist:** Stand up and slowly reach over and touch your toes as you bend at the waist. Try to keep your knees straight. Repeat 10 times.
    Remain standing up and spread your legs apart about two feet. Bend to the left side at the waist, reaching your right

arm over your head. Repeat 5 times and then repeat this exercise bending on your right side with your left arm over your head.

Exercise 3: Muscle Tension Release, Energy Level Increase

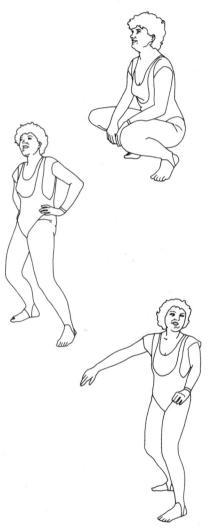

This exercise set is excellent for releasing muscle tension, improving circulation, and increasing your energy. You may have a feeling of vigor and vitality upon completing this set. The pelvic movements are particularly helpful in bringing optimal blood flow, oxygen, and nutrients to this region, which may help menopause problems such as atrophic vaginitis and hot flashes.

As your strength and flexibility improve, you may want to do the steps a little more vigorously. At the beginning, however, do the steps slowly and *never* do them so hard as to cause a strain or injury.

1. **Legs and Pelvis:** Stand with your legs spread apart about two feet. Point your feet out at a comfortable angle. Bend your knees slowly and lower your buttocks. Eventually, they should be able to go as low as your knees. Move up and down 10 times.

2. **Legs and Pelvis:** Stand with your legs spread about two feet with feet facing forward. Rock your pelvis back and forth. Repeat 10 times.

3. **Legs and Pelvis:** Move your hips and pelvis from side to side. Let your torso and arms sway in the opposite direction, as if dancing.

4. **Entire Body** (especially trunk, abdomen, and extremities): Jump up and down in place for several minutes. Allow your

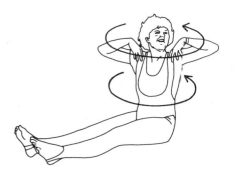

arms to move freely up and down. Shake out your wrists, and raise your arms over your head while you jump to release tension in the shoulders and arms.

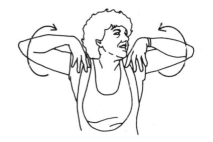

5. **Shoulders, Neck, Torso:** Sit down with your legs out in front. Raise your arms to shoulder level, bending at the elbow. Place your hands on your shoulders with your fingers in front and thumb in back. Turn your elbows, head, and neck to the left and then to the right. Repeat 10 times. Be sure to let your entire torso move with your shoulders and arms.

   Move your shoulders in circles in a forward direction 10 times. Repeat in circles in a backward direction 10 times. Allow your torso to follow the shoulders so the movement is fluid.

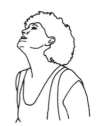

6. **Neck and Head:** Still remaining in a sitting position, flex your neck downward so that your face looks at the floor. Then extend your neck up so your face looks at the ceiling. Repeat slowly 10 times. Then turn your head from side to side (left to right). Repeat 10 times.

7. **Eyes:** From a sitting position, look straight ahead. Then slowly raise your eyes up and down, then side to side. Repeat 10 times.

Books

Cailliet, Rene, M.D., and Leonard Gross. *The Rejuvenation Strategy*. New York: Pocket Books, 1987.

Columbo, Franco, D.C., and Anita Columbu, D.C. *Starbodies, The Women's Weight Training Book*. New York: E.P. Dutton, 1978.

Goldman, Bob, and Ronald Klatz. *The "E" Factor*. New York: Morrow, 1988.

Jerome, John. *Staying Supple*. New York: Bantam Books, 1987.

Leen, Edie. *The Complete Women's Weight Training Guide*. New York: Macmillan, 1980.

McLish, Rachel, and Vedral Joyce, Ph.D., *Perfect Parts*. New York: Warner Books, 1987.

Pinkney, Callan. *Callanetics: 10 Years Younger in 10 Hours*. New York: Avon, 1984.

Principal, Victoria. *The Body Principal*. New York: Simon & Schuster, 1983.

Tobias, Maxine, and Mary Stewart. *Stretch and Relax*. Tucson, Az.: The Body Press, 1985.

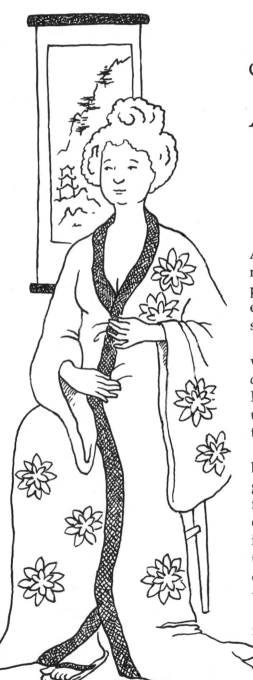

CHAPTER 13

Acupressure Massage

Acupressure is a traditional therapy developed by the Chinese many centuries ago. It is an easy-to-use method of applying finger pressure to specific points on the body that can help to prevent disease and illness. Acupressure can be very helpful in relieving the symptoms of menopause as well as problems related to aging.

This treatment method is based on the belief that there exists within the body a life energy or "biofield." This life energy is called *chi*. It is different from, yet similar to electromagnetic energy. Health is thought to be a state in which the chi is equally distributed throughout the body and is present in sufficient amounts. It is thought to energize all the cells and tissues of the body.

This life energy is thought to be distributed throughout the body by channels called meridians. This distribution system is analogous to blood and lymph vessels, except that the latter distribute fluid and the meridians distribute a subtle energy. Meridians move energy through the body like invisible rivers flowing deep into the interior of the body through the organ systems and at times along the skin surface. The place where the energy surfaces on the skin is called the acupuncture point. The electrical resistance of the skin at these points is slightly different from that of the surrounding skin.

Disease is thought to occur when the energy flow through a meridian stops or is blocked. Then the internal organ system that corresponds to the meridian manifests symptoms of disease. The meridian flow can be corrected by stimulating the points on the skin surface. These points can be treated either by hand massage, insertion of needles, or by electrical stimulus. When the normal flow of energy through the body is resumed, the body is believed to heal itself spontaneously.

Stimulation of the acupressure points can be used to help relieve menopause symptoms. The simplest and most effective way is to use finger pressure. This can be done by you or by a friend following simple instructions. It is safe, painless, and does not require the use of needles. It can be used without the years of specialized training needed for insertion of needles.

I have used acupressure on my patients for many problems including premenstrual tension, headaches, and muscle strains, as well as for menopause symptoms. I have seen acupressure work on stubborn and resistant cases where nothing else seemed to be effective.

How to Perform Acupressure

1. Acupressure should be done either on yourself or by a friend when you are relaxed. Your room should be warm and quiet. Hands should be clean and nails trimmed to avoid bruising yourself. If your hands are cold, put them under warm water.

2. Choose the side of the body to work on that has the most discomfort. For example, you may have a cyst in one breast. Work the points on that side of the body. If both sides are equally uncomfortable, choose whichever one you want. Working on one side seems to relieve the symptoms on both sides. There appears to be a transfer of energy or information from one side to the other.

3. Hold each point indicated in the exercise with a steady pressure for one to three minutes. Pressure should be applied slowly with the tips or balls of the fingers. It is best to place several fingers over the area of the point. If you feel resistance

or tension in the area on which you are applying pressure, you may want to push a little harder. However, if your hand starts to feel tense or tired, lighten the pressure a bit. Make sure that your hand is comfortable. The acupressure point may feel somewhat tender. This means that the energy pathway or meridian is blocked.

4. During the treatment, the tenderness in the point should slowly go away. You may also have a subjective feeling of energy radiating from this point into the body. Many patients describe this sensation as very pleasant. Don't worry if you don't feel it—not everyone does. The main goal is relief from your symptoms.

5. Breathe gently while doing each exercise.

6. The point that you are to hold is shown in the photograph accompanying the exercise. All of these points correspond to specific points on the acupressure meridians.

7. You may massage the points once a day or more during the time that you have symptoms.

The Exercises

Acupressure Exercise 1:
General Balancing of the Energy Pathways

This sequence of points balances the energy flow of the entire body and benefits many of the meridians. These points stimulate vigor and vitality and improve the overall health of the body. They are a good sequence to perform before doing the specific corrective points for female health problems.

1. Hold each step for 1 to 3 minutes.

2. Lie on your stomach.
   Left hand holds point above your pubic bone and below your navel.
   Right hand is placed over left hand.

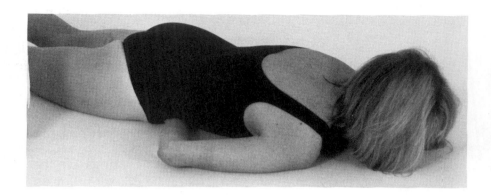

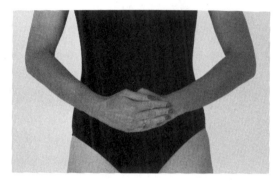

This photograph shows correct placement of hands.

3. Turn over and lie on your back.
   Place both hands beneath your lower back.
   Make a fist with both hands. Press fist into the thick ropelike muscles of your lower back.

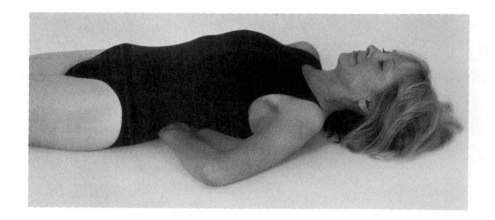

4. Sit upright on a chair.
   Bend your right arm at the elbow joint.
   Left hand holds point about one inch below the crease of the right elbow toward your hand.

5. Sit upright on a chair.
   Place your right hand in your lap. Left hand holds point 1½ inches from the wrist crease on the back of the right hand.

6. Sit upright on a chair.
   Left hand holds the point on the tip of the shoulder, midway between the outside of the neck and the outside of the shoulders. The point is slightly to the back.

7. Sit upright on a chair.
   Left hand holds the point between the eyebrows.

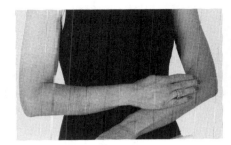

4.

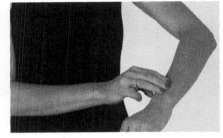

5.

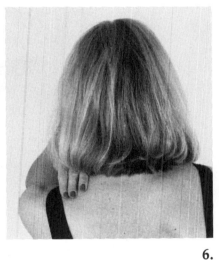

6.

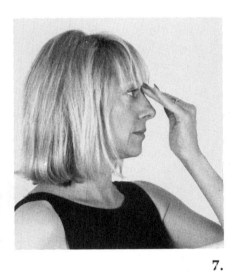

7.

Exercise 2: Balances the Entire Reproductive Tract

This exercise alleviates all menstrual and menopause complaints, balances the energy of the female reproductive tract, and relieves lower back pain and abdominal discomfort. It is helpful for the control of excessive menstrual bleeding and hot flashes.

Equipment. This exercise uses a knotted hand towel to put pressure on hard-to-reach areas of the back. Place the knotted towel on these points while your two hands are on the other points. This increases your ability to unblock the energy pathways of your body.

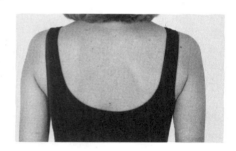

1. Lie on the floor with your knees up as you lie down. Place the towel between the shoulder blades on the spine. Hold each step 1 to 3 minutes.

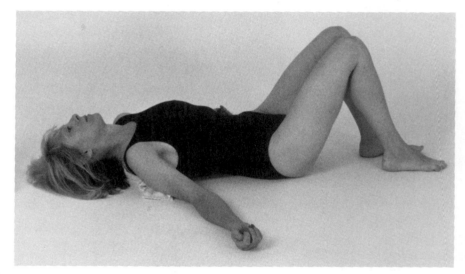

2. Cross your arms on your chest. Press your thumbs against the right and left inside arms.

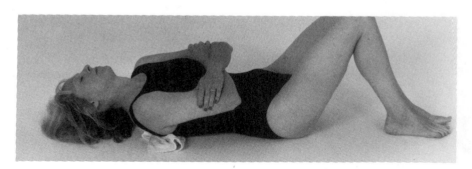

3. Left hand holds point at the base of the sternum (breastbone).
  Right hand holds point at the base of the head (at the junction of the spine and the skull).

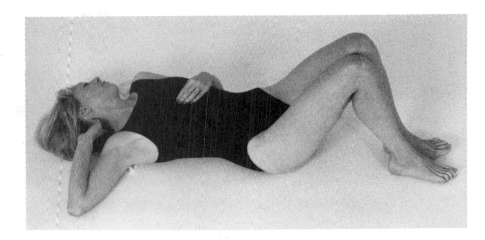

4. Interlace fingers. Place them below your breasts. Fingertips should press directly against the body.

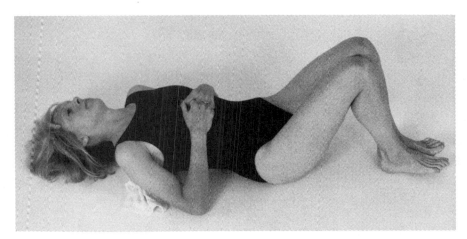

5. Move the knotted towel along the spine to the waistline.

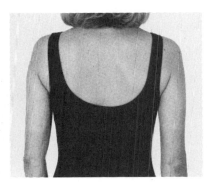

6. Left hand should be placed
at the top of the pubic bone,
pressing down.
　　Right hand holds point on
tailbone.

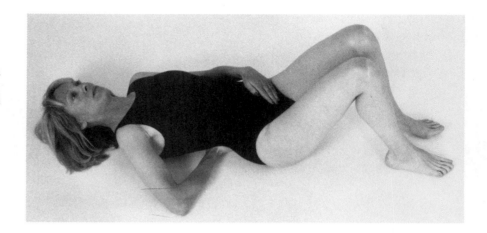

Exercise 3: Relieves Lower Back Pain and Cramps

　　This exercise normalizes the energy of the reproductive organs
by balancing points on the bladder meridian. It also relieves lower
back pain.

1. Sit on the floor and prop
your back against a wall or a
heavy piece of furniture.
Hold each step 1 to 3
minutes.

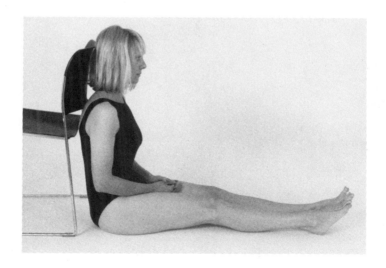

Alternative Method: Lie on the floor and put your lower legs over the seat of a chair. Follow the exercise from that position.

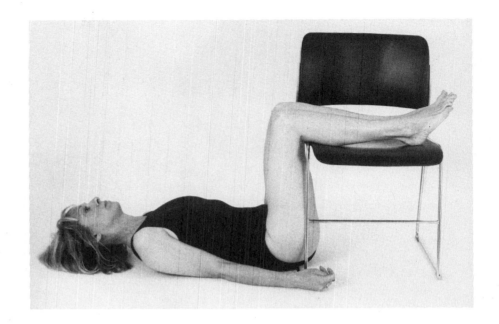

2. Place left hand 1 inch above the waist on the muscle to the left side of the spine (muscle will feel firm and ropelike).

Place right hand behind crease of the left knee.

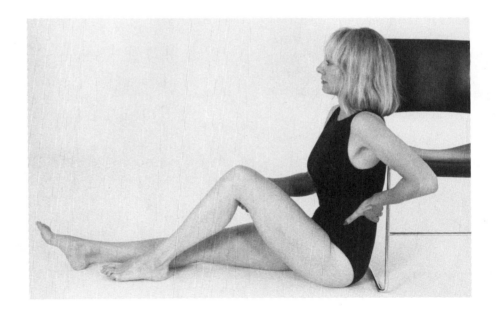

3. Left hand stays in the same position.

Right hand is placed on the center of the back of the left calf. This is just below the fullest part of the calf.

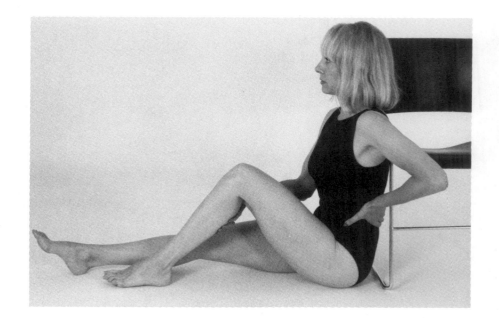

4. Left hand remains 1 inch above the waist on the muscle to the side of the spine.

Right hand is placed just below the ankle bone on the outside of the left heel.

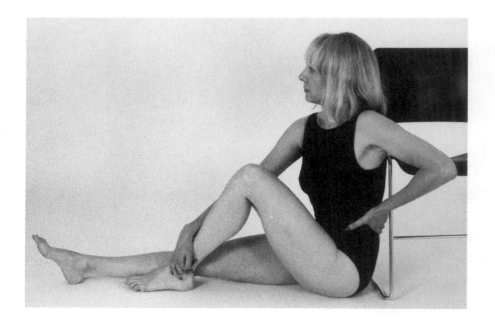

5. Left hand remains 1 inch above the waist on the muscle to the side of the spine.

Right hand holds the front and back of the left little toenail.

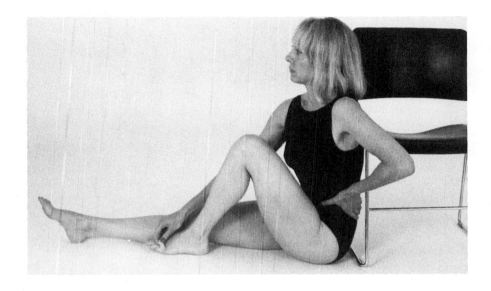

Exercise 4: Relieves Excessive Menstrual Bleeding

This exercise is useful in controlling excessive uterine bleeding, which is common as women approach menopause.

1. Sit upright on a chair. Hold each step for 1 to 3 minutes.

Bend over at waist with right hand holding point in front of ankle bone. Move hand slowly along points on leg.

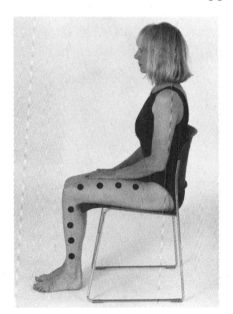
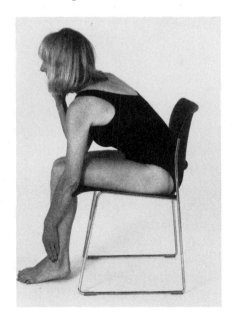

2. Move right hand slowly on points to the top of the thigh.
    Repeat on other side with left hand.

3. Right hand in middle of thigh points up to groin. Repeat on other side with left hand. Circle area around navel in counterclockwise direction.

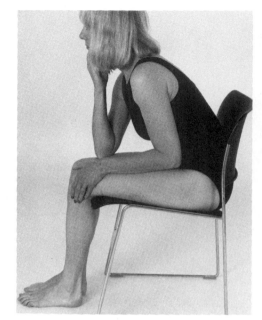

2.

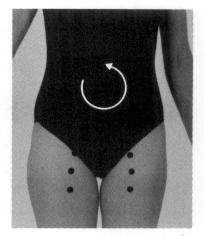

3.

Exercise 5: Relieves Menopause Symptoms and Thyroid Imbalances

This exercise is useful for relief of hot flashes and energizes the thyroid.

1. Sit upright on a chair. Hold each step for 1 to 3 minutes. Hands wrap around shoulders with thumbs pressing gently into both sides on top of collarbone.

2. Fingers are in back and press against upper shoulders and shoulder blade area.

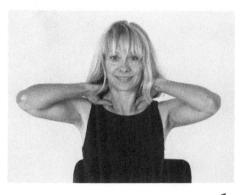

1.   2.

Exercise 6: Relieves Hot Flashes

This exercise relieves hot flashes.

1. Sit on the floor with the knees bent. Hold each step 1 to 3 minutes. Right hand holds point below little toe.

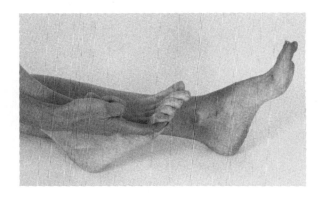

2. Right hand holds point above middle toe. Then, hand moves to point behind ankle bone.

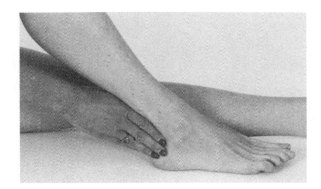

3. Left hand holds point on right hand on outside of 4th finger.
   Repeat sequence on left side.

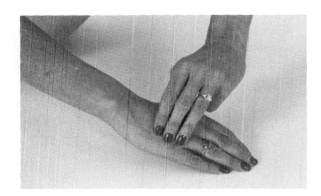

Exercise 7: Relieves Hot Flashes and Skin Disorders

This exercise relieves hot flashes and is excellent for various skin problems.

1. Sit on the floor with the knees bent. Hold each step 1 to 3 minutes.

2. Left hand holds left calf.
   Right hand holds right calf.

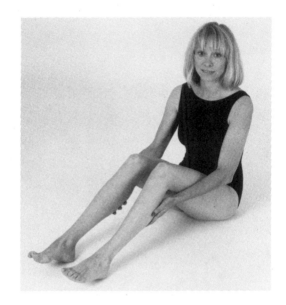

3. Cross arms. Left hand holds right calf.
   Right hand holds left calf.

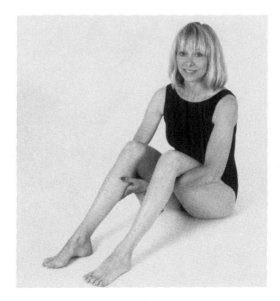

Exercise 8: Relieves Atrophic Vaginitis

This exercise relieves the symptoms of atrophic vaginitis commonly seen during menopause by relieving insufficient vaginal lubrication.

1. Sit on the floor with the knees bent. Hold each step 1 to 3 minutes. Right hand holds point in the middle of sole of foot. (Do not use this point in pregnancy.)

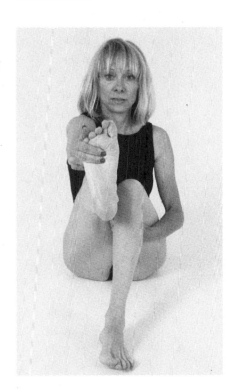

2. Right hand moves to point behind ankle bone. Repeat this sequence on left side.

3. Right hand moves to point above the bladder in the midline of the body.

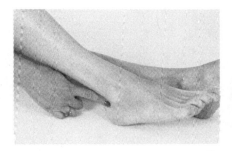

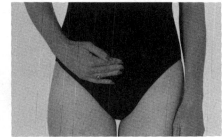

2.

3.

Exercise 9: Relieves Atrophic Vaginitis

This exercise relieves atrophic vaginitis by promoting vaginal tone.

1. Sit on floor with knees bent. Hold each step 1 to 3 minutes. Right hand holds point in middle of sole of foot. (Do not use this point in pregnancy.)

2. Right hand moves to point below little toe.

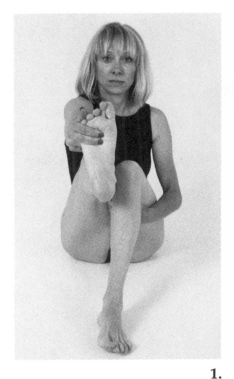

1.

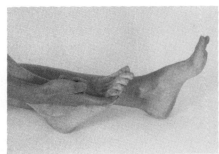

2.

3. Right hand then moves to point behind ankle bone. Repeat this sequence on left side.

4. Right hand moves to point in pubic area on right and left side.

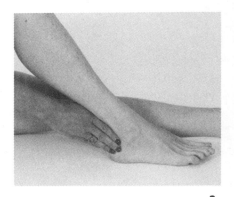

3.

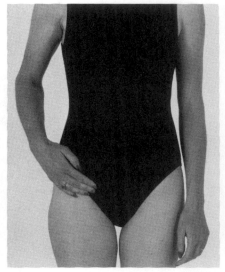

4.

Exercise 10: Relieves Lack of Sexual Desire

This exercise helps to stimulate sexual desire and helps to relieve frigidity.

Equipment. This exercise uses a knotted hand towel to put pressure on hard-to-reach areas of the back. Place the knotted towel on these points while your two hands are on the other points. This increases your ability to unblock the energy pathways of your body.

1. Lie down on the floor. Hold each step for 1 to 3 minutes. Place knotted towel under the right shoulder blade; left fist is under right waist. Right hand holds left inner thigh.

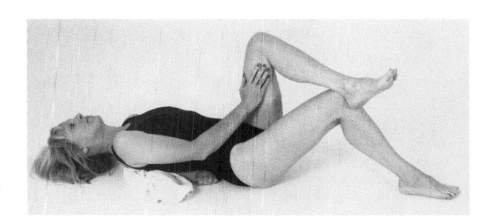

2. Left hand under tailbone, right hand holds pubic bone.

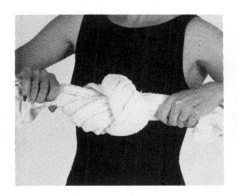

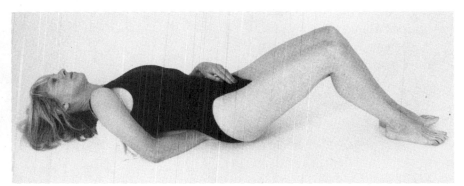

3. Left hand stays under tail-bone, right hand presses left groin.
   Repeat sequence on other side.

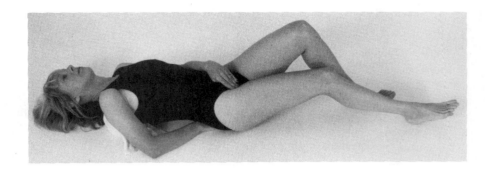

Exercise 11: Relieves Symptoms of Bladder Problems

This exercise promotes bladder health. Bladder tissues often become thin and weak with menopause.

1. Sit on the floor with knees bent. Hold each point for 1 to 3 minutes. Right hand on point below little toe.

2. Right hand moves to point on foot above little toe.
   Repeat this sequence on the opposite side.

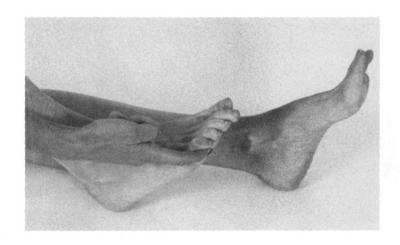

Exercise 12: Relieves Nervous Tension, Insomnia

This exercise helps to promote sleep and reduces nervous tension.

1. Lie on the floor. Hold each step for 1 to 3 minutes. Place right hand in the hollow in front of the neck. Place left hand on the pubic bone.

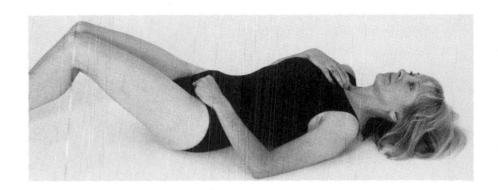

Exercise 13: Relieves Depression, Headaches, Tightness of Neck and Shoulders, and Hypoglycemia

The neck and shoulders generally carry a great deal of tension. Tightness in this area can act as a bottleneck and can impede the energy flow of the entire body. Thus, the entire body is energized by this exercise. It also relieves depression.

A major treatment point for hypoglycemia is worked on in this exercise. This may help reduce the excessive cravings for sweets that some women suffer from.

1. Sit comfortably or lie down. Hold each step 1 to 3 minutes.

2. Left hand holds point at the top of the shoulder blade, 1 to 2 inches to the side of the spine. The point is between the shoulder blade and the spine. It may feel firm and resistant.

   Right hand holds the same point on the right side.

3. Left hand holds points slightly to the back of the top of the shoulder where the neck meets the shoulder.

   Right hand holds the same point on the right side.

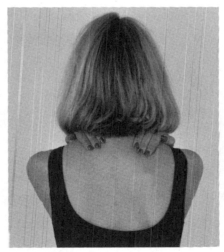

2.

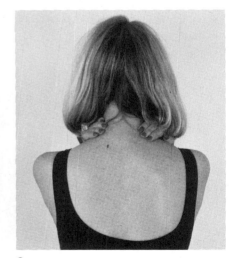

3.

4. Left hand holds the point halfway up the neck, fingers sit on the muscle next to the spine.

   Right hand holds the same point on the right side.

5. Left hand holds the point at the base of the skull 1 to 2 inches from the spine.

   Right hand holds the same point on the right side.

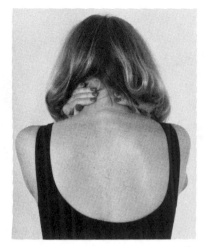

4.

Exercise 14: Promotes Healthy Bones

This exercise is useful in helping to prevent osteoporosis.

1. Sit on the floor with knees bent. Hold each step for 1 to 3 minutes. Right hand holds point in middle of sole of foot (do not use this point during pregnancy).

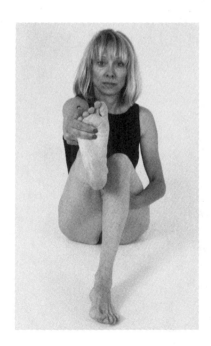

2. Right hand moves to the point below little toe.

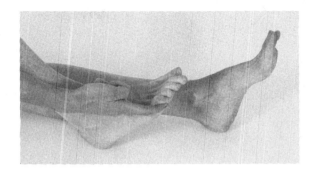

3. Right hand moves to point behind ankle bone.
   Repeat this sequence on left side.

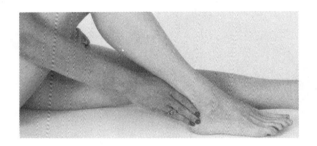

Exercise 15: Relieves Fibrocystic Breast Problems and Promotes Breast Health

This exercise helps to promote healthy breasts.

1. Sit on the floor. Hold each point for 1 to 3 minutes.

2. Both hands move over points around breast in outward direction.

3. Right hand moves to points in pubic area.

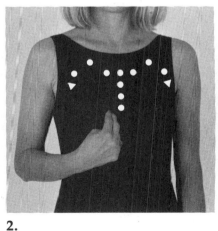

2.

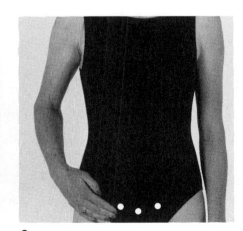

3.

4. Right hand moves up leg to shin.

5. Left hand moves up points on right arm above wrist toward elbow.
    Repeat sequence on opposite side.

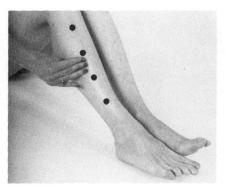

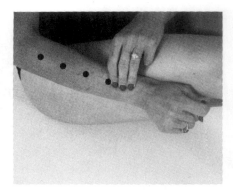

4.   5.

The Right Exercise for Your Symptoms

The preceding exercises may be useful for each category of menopause symptoms. All of the exercises listed for each symptom group in the Complete Treatment Chart on pages 32–35 and in the abbreviated chart below can be helpful.

In the beginning, try all those that pertain to your symptoms. You may find that you enjoy certain ones more than others. It is only by trial and error that you will find the ones that bring you the most relief.

Acupressure Exercises for Menopause Symptoms

Symptoms	Acupressure Exercise
Entire female reproductive tract	1, 2, 3
Irregular heavy bleeding (Menorrhagia)	2, 3, 4
Hot flashes	2, 5, 6, 7
Atrophic vaginitis	2, 3, 8, 9
Sexual desire, relieve frigidity	2, 10

Symptoms	Acupressure Exercise
Bladder, lower urinary tract	2, 3, 10, 11
Anxiety, irritability, insomnia	1, 12
Depression, fatigue	13
Osteoporosis	14
Breast problems	15
Thyroid problems	2, 13
Pelvic organs	2, 3

Suggested Reading for Acupressure:

The Academy of Traditional Chinese Medicine. *An Outline of Chinese Acupuncture*. New York: Pergamon Press, 1975.

Bauer, Cathryn. *Acupressure for Women*. Freedom, Ca.: The Crossing Press, 1987.

Chang, Stephen Thomas. *The Complete Book of Acupuncture*. Berkeley, Ca.: Celestial Arts, 1976.

Gach, Michael Reed. *The Bum Back Book*. Berkeley, Ca.: Celestial Arts, 1983.

Gach, Michael Reed, and Carolyn Marco. *Acu-Yoga*. Tokyo: Japan Publications, 1981.

Houston, F. M. *The Healing Benefits of Acupressure*. New Canaan, Ct.: Keats Publishing, 1974.

Kenyon, Julian. *Acupressure Techniques*. Rochester, Vt.: Healing Arts Press, 1980.

Nickel, David J. *Acupressure for Athletes*. New York: Henry Holt, 1984.

Pendleton, Bonnie, and Betty Mehling. *Relax/With Self-Therap/Ease*. Englewood Cliffs, N.J.: Prentice-Hall, 1984.

Teeguarden, Iona. *Acupressure Way of Health: Jin Shin Do*. Tokyo: Japan Publications, 1978.

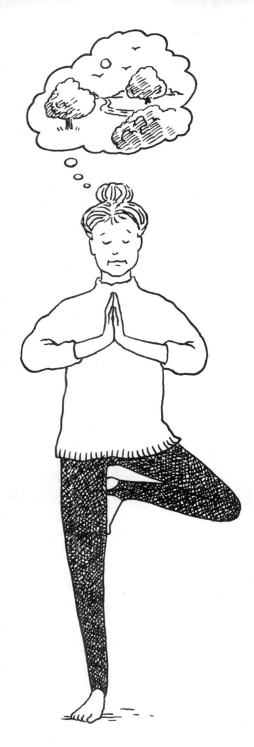

CHAPTER 14

Yoga for Menopause

Yoga originated thousands of years ago in India as a system of physical exercises combined with deep breathing and meditation. The traditional goal of yoga was to promote balance and harmony in the practitioner. Done properly, the exercises promote health on all levels—physical, mental, emotional, and spiritual.

Hatha Yoga is the type most commonly taught in the United States. It is based on physical exercises called *asanas* and breathing exercises called *pranayamas*. The effects of the yoga stretches on menopause and other problems of aging may be extremely helpful when combined with proper nutrition and other lifestyle habits.

The poses in this chapter will gently stretch every muscle in your body and will energize and balance the female reproductive tract, breasts, thyroid, and endocrine system. They are also helpful for problems of the digestive tract, nervous system, circulation, and all other organ systems of the body. I personally do yoga stretches every other day as part of my exercise routine. I find that they increase my vigor and stamina and help me to maintain muscle and joint flexibility.

When doing the exercises, it is important that you focus and concentrate on the positions. First your mind visualizes how the exercise is to look, and then your body follows with the correct placement of the pose. The exercises are done through slow, controlled stretching movements. This slowness allows you to have greater control over your body movements. You minimize the possibility of injury and maximize the benefit to the particular part of the body to which your attention is being directed.

How to Perform Yoga for Menopause

1. Yoga should be performed in a relaxed and unhurried manner. Be sure to set aside adequate time, between 10 to 30 minutes, so that you do not feel rushed. Your work area should be quiet, peaceful, and uncluttered.

2. Choose a flat area and work on a mat or a blanket. This will make you more comfortable while you do the exercises.

3. Wear loose, comfortable clothing. It is better that you work without socks to give your feet complete freedom of movement and to prevent slipping.

4. Evacuate your bowels or bladder before you begin the exercises. Wait at least two hours after eating to exercise.

5. Try to practice these movements on a regular basis. Every day for a few minutes is best, particularly when you have menopause symptoms. If that is not possible, then try to practice them every other day.

6. Pay close attention to the initial instructions when beginning an exercise. Look at the placement of the body as shown in the photographs. This is very important, for if the pose is practiced properly, you are much more likely to have relief of your symptoms.

7. Try to visualize the pose in your mind, then follow with proper placement of the body.

8. Move slowly through the pose. This will help promote flexibility of the muscles and prevent injury.

9. Follow the breathing instructions provided in the exercise. Most important, do not hold your breath. Always allow your

breathing to flow. It is important that you time your breathing with the placement of the body position.

10. Always rest for a few minutes after doing yoga stretches.

11. Don't be discouraged if you can't do as much as the model in the photos. The model represents the optimal position. If you practice regularly in a slow, unhurried fashion you will gradually loosen your muscles, ligaments, and joints. You may be surprised at how supple you can become over time. If you experience any pain or discomfort you have probably overreached your current ability and should immediately reduce the amount of the stretching until you can proceed without discomfort. Be careful, as muscular injuries can take quite a while to heal. If you do strain a muscle, I have found that immediately applying ice to the injured area for 10 minutes is quite helpful. Continue to use the ice pack 2 to 3 times a day for several days. If the pain persists, see your doctor.

Stretch 1: The Pump

This exercise strengthens the back and abdominal muscles, improves blood circulation to the pelvic organs, and calms anxiety and nervousness.

1. Lie down and press the small of your back to the floor. This permits you to use your abdominal muscles without straining your lower back.

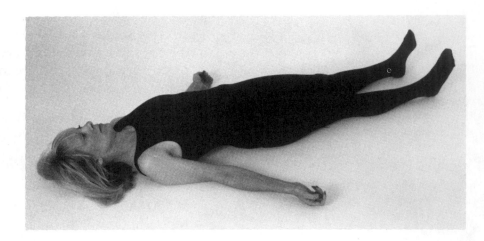

2. Raise your right leg slowly while breathing in. Keep your back flat on the floor and let the rest of your body remain relaxed. Move your leg very slowly; imagine your leg being pulled up smoothly by a spring. Do not move your leg in a jerking manner. Hold for a few breaths. Lower your leg and breathe out.

3. Repeat the same exercise on your left side. Then alternate legs, repeating the exercise 5 to 10 times.

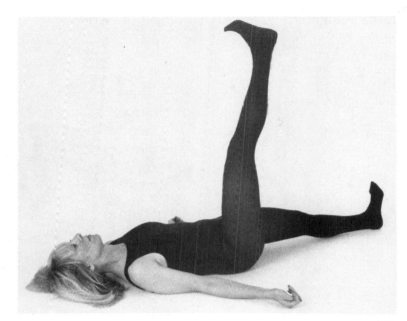

2.

Stretch 2: Spinal Flex

This exercise emphasizes freer pelvic movement with controlled breathing, energizes and rejuvenates the female reproductive tract, and tones the abdominal organs (pancreas, liver, and adrenals). It may even have benefits for skin health.

1. Lie on your back with your knees bent and your feet on the floor close to your buttocks.

2. Exhale and press the lower back to the floor, raising the buttocks slightly.

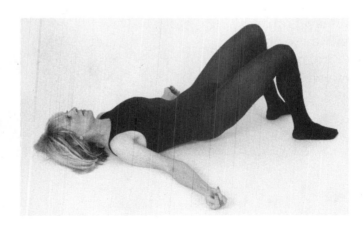

3. Arch the back slightly.

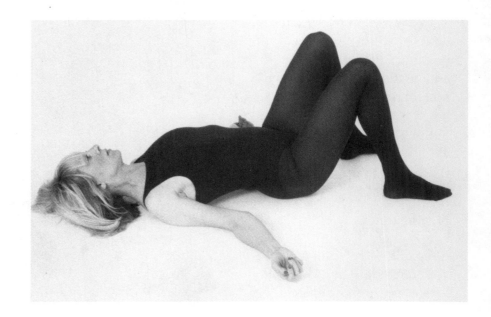

4. Inhale and lift your lower back from the floor. This stretches the region from the sternum to the pelvis.

5. Repeat this exercise 10 times. Always lift your navel up on the in-breath. Always elongate your spine and press the lower back down on the out-breath.

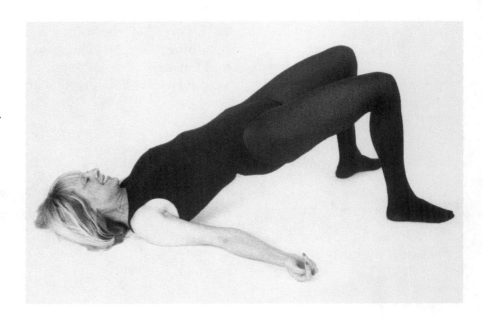

Stretch 3: The Locust

This exercise energizes the entire female reproductive tract, thyroid, liver, intestines, and kidneys. It can also help relieve menopause symptoms. It strengthens the lower back, abdomen, buttocks and legs, and prevents lower back pain, and also helps to reduce weight in the thighs and hips, and tightens and firms the skin in these areas.

1. Lie face down on the floor. Make fists with both hands and place them under your hips. This prevents compression of the lumbar spine while doing the exercise.

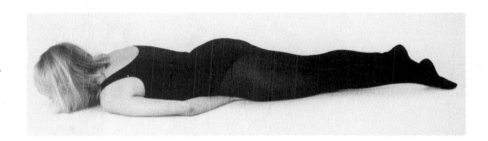

2. Straighten your body and raise your right leg with an upward thrust as high as you can, keeping your hips on your fists. Hold for 5 to 20 seconds if possible.

3. Lower the leg and slowly return to your original position. Repeat on the left side, then with both legs together. Remember to keep your hips resting on your fists.

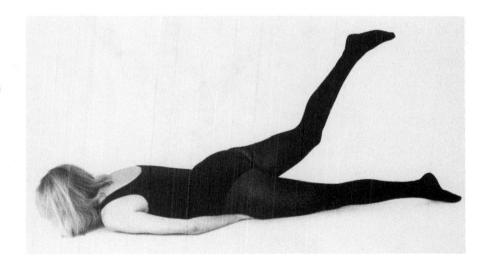

Stretch 4: Wide-Angle Pose

This exercise opens the entire pelvic region, energizes the female reproductive tract, and may help relieve menopause symptoms. It is helpful for varicose veins and improves circulation in the legs.

1. Lie on your back, with your legs against the wall and extended out like a V or an arc, and your arms extended to the side. Hips should be as close to the wall as possible, buttocks on the floor. Legs should be spread apart as far as they can and still remain comfortable. Breathing easily, hold for 1 minute, allowing the inner thighs to relax.

2. Bring legs together and hold for 1 minute.

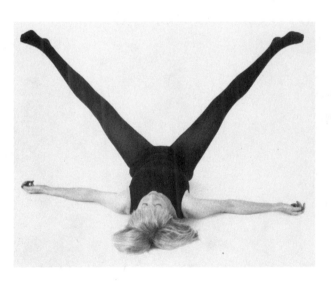
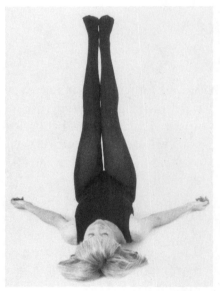

Stretch 5: The Plow

This exercise improves circulation to the brain and may help relieve hot flashes and other menopause symptoms. It also reduces swelling and fluid retention in the legs and ankles. It stimulates the thyroid, improves the elasticity of the spine, strengthens the back, and relaxes the abdomen and neck. It helps to reduce weight in the hips, thighs, legs, and abdomen.

1. Put a chair on your mat. Lie on your back, facing upward, away from the chair. Arms are at your sides and palms are facing downward so that they press against the floor. Legs should be together.

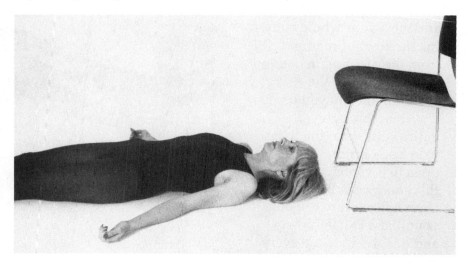

2. Slowly raise your legs and hips over your head until your toes touch the chair. This should be done without jerking, so bend your knees if necessary. (This exercise is usually done by bringing the legs and hips over the head until the toes touch the floor, but bringing the feet all the way to the floor could be harmful for women with menopause, since they often have a concavity of the back.) Lift the spine by stretching the back muscles as much as possible. This exercise will alleviate compression of the lumbar spine.

3. To come out of this posture, bend your knees and roll down slowly onto your back. Return to your original position.

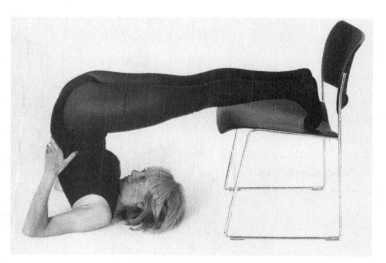

Stretch 6: The Sponge

This exercise relieves anxiety and irritability and reduces eye tension and swelling of the face. It is a helpful exercise before going to bed if you have menopause insomnia.

1. Lie on your back. Your arms should be at your sides, palms up. Close your eyes and relax your whole body. Inhale slowly, breathing from the diaphragm. As you inhale, visualize the energy in the air around you being drawn in through your entire body. Imagine that your body is porous and open like a sponge so that this energy can be drawn in to revitalize every cell of your body. Exhale slowly and deeply, allowing every ounce of tension to be drained from your body.

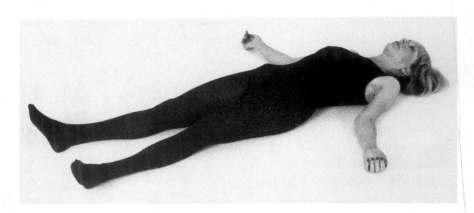

Stretch 7: Child's Pose

This exercise is excellent for calming menopause anxiety and irritability. It gently stretches the lower back.

1. Sit on your heels. Bring your forehead to the floor, stretching the spine as far over your head as possible. Close your eyes. Hold for as long as this is comfortable.

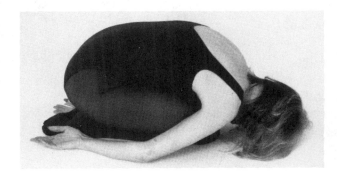

Stretch 8: Upward Facing Dog

This exercise elevates mood and can help to relieve depression. It also relieves lower back pain and strengthens the spine. It improves blood circulation to the pelvic region and encourages chest expansion and lung elasticity.

1. Lie on the floor on your stomach, head facing downward. Place your palms on the floor under your shoulders, fingers pointing straight ahead.

2. As you inhale, raise your head and trunk, stretching your spine forward and curving it into a gentle C. Make sure your elbows are straight. Avoid hunching up your shoulders. Hips and knees lift off the floor. Legs are straight and heels press back to help stretch the spine. The weight of the body will rest only on the hands and toes. Hold the pose 30 seconds to 1 minute, breathing deeply. Spine, thighs, and calves should be fully stretched and the buttocks contracted.

3. Bend your elbows, releasing the stretch. Return to the original position and rest for a minute.

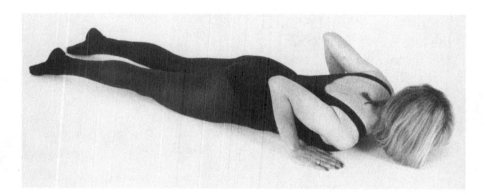

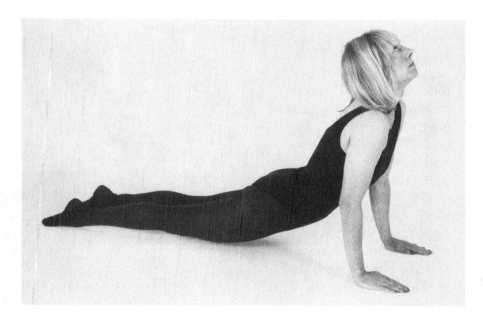

Stretch 9: The Bow

This exercise relieves menopause depression, fatigue, and lethargy, improving your energy and elevating your mood.

1. Lie down on the floor, arms at your sides.
   Slowly bend your legs at the knees and bring your feet up toward your buttocks. Reach back with your arms and carefully take hold of one foot and then the other. Flex your feet to make grasping them easier.

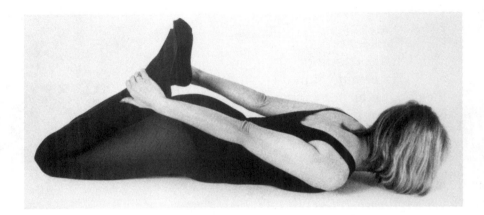

2. Inhale and raise your trunk from the floor as far as possible. Lift your head and bring your knees as close together and as close to the floor as possible. Squeeze the buttocks. Imagine your body looking like a gently curved bow. Hold for 10 to 15 seconds. Tying your knees together with a soft tie may help you do this exercise.

3. Slowly release the pose. Allow your chin to touch the floor and finally release your feet and return them slowly to the floor. Return to your original position.

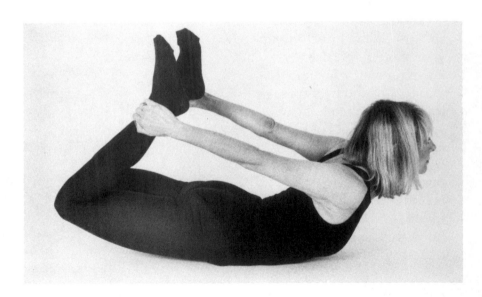

Stretch 10: Chest Expander

This exercise improves circulation to the upper half of the body and energizes and stimulates it. It also loosens and stretches tense muscles in the upper body, especially the shoulders, chest, and back. It expands the lungs and energizes the breasts and heart.

1. Stand easily. Arms should be at your sides, feet are hip distance apart.

2. Extend your arms forward until your palms touch.

3. Bring your arms back slowly and gracefully until you can clasp them behind your back. Exhale, then straighten your clasped hands and arms as far as you can without discomfort. Remember to stand upright; body should not bend forward. Breathe deeply.

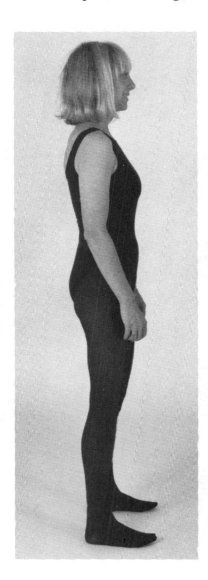 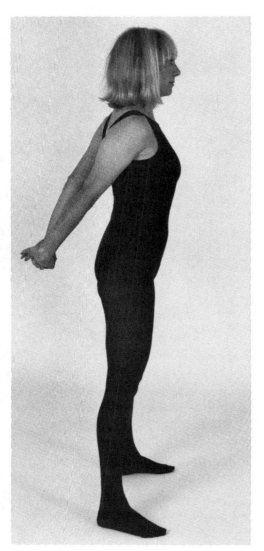

4. Inhale deeply and bend backward from the waist. Keep your hands clasped and your arms held high. Drop your head backward a few inches and look upward as you relax your shoulders and the back of your neck. Hold this position for a few seconds.

5. As you hold your breath, bend forward at the waist, bringing your clasped hands and arms up over your back. Relax your neck muscles and keep your knees straight. Hold for a few seconds.

6. Exhale as you return to the upright position. Unclasp your hands and allow your arms to rest easily at your sides. Repeat entire sequence 3 times.

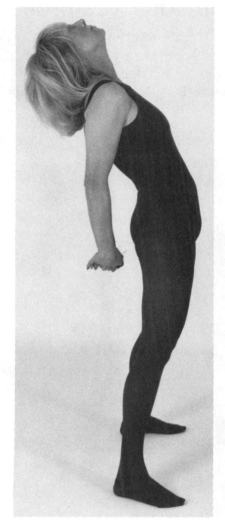

4.

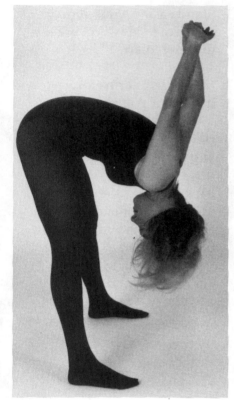

5.

Stretch 11: Lion

This exercise stimulates the thyroid, neck area, and throat.

1. Sit on your knees with your hands on your thighs. Take in a deep breath and stretch your body upward. As you exhale, widen eyes, stick out your tongue with intensity, and push the body forward. Hold this position until the count of 10. Repeat this exercise 5 times.

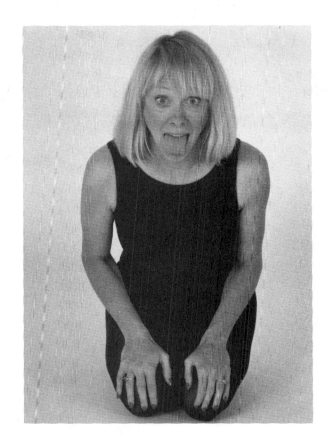

Stretch 12: Tree

This exercise improves concentration and awareness. It also improves balance and posture.

1. Stand erect and focus your eyes on a stationary point. Place one foot against opposite inner thigh so that one leg is bearing the weight. Slowly raise arms. Hold for a count of 5. Reverse sides. Repeat 3 times.

   Note: You may place one hand on the wall for support if needed.

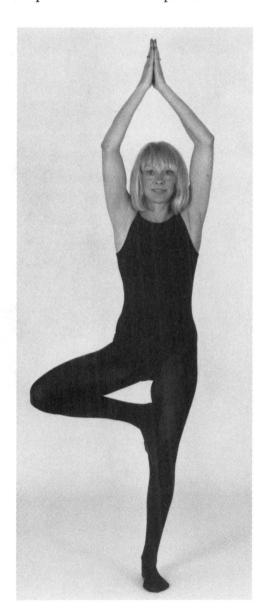

The Right Stretch for Your Symptoms

The preceding exercises may be useful for menopause and other problems of aging. Prior to doing the specific correctives, it is recommended that you spend the first week or two of your program doing the general flexibility and fitness exercises in the chapter on exercise. They are meant to tone and improve flexibility of your entire body. Determine which warmups you enjoy the most and practice them on a regular basis, either daily or every other day.

Beginning on week 2 or 3, they can be followed by the specific correctives for menopause and other problems. For your convenience, the exercises are listed here according to the symptoms they relieve.

- Entire female reproductive tract: Pump, Spinal Flex, Locust, Wide-Angle Pose, Upward Facing Dog.
- Hot flashes: Pump, Spinal Flex, Locust, Wide-Angle Pose, Upward Facing Dog.
- Atrophic vaginitis: Pump, Spinal Flex, Locust, Wide-Angle Pose, Upward Facing Dog.
- Sexual desire, frigidity: Pump, Spinal Flex, Locust, Wide-Angle Pose, Upward Facing Dog.
- Bladder, lower urinary tract changes: Pump, Spinal Flex, Locust, Wide-Angle Pose, Upward Facing Dog.
- Psychological symptoms—anxiety, irritability, insomnia: Pump, Sponge, Child's Pose.
- Psychological symptoms—depression, fatigue: Upward Facing Dog, Bow
- Osteoporosis: Pump, Spinal Flex, Locust, Wide-Angle Pose, Plow, Bow, Upward Facing Dog, Chest Expander, Lion, Tree
- Breast health, prevention of disease: Upward Facing Dog, Chest Expander
- Thyroid health, prevention of disease: Locust, Plow, Lion
- Pelvic organs, prevention of disease: Pump, Spinal Flex, Locust, Wide-Angle Pose, Upward Facing Dog

Suggested Reading for Yoga:

Bell, Lorna, and Endora Seyfer. *Gentle Yoga*. Berkeley Ca.: Celestial Arts, 1987.

Couch, Jean, and Nell Weaver. *Runner's World Yoga Book*. New York: Runner's World Books, 1979.

Moore, Marcia, and Mark Douglas. *Yoga*. Arcane, Me.: Arcane Publications, 1967.

Singh, Ravi, *Kundalini Yoga*. New York: White Lion Press, 1988.

Stearn, Jess. *Yoga, Youth and Reincarnation*. New York: Bantam, 1965.

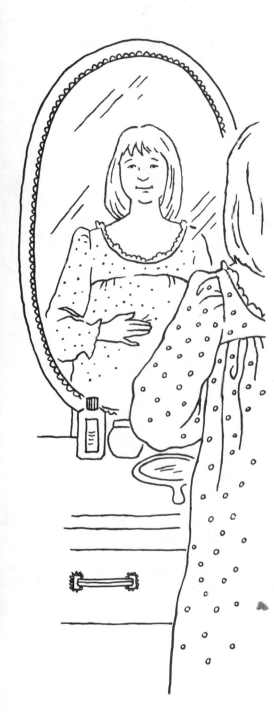

CHAPTER 15

Neurovascular and Neurolymphatic Holding Points

Neurolymphatic Massage Points

The lymphatics are the drainage system of the body. They consist of tiny vessels that carry waste products from the periphery of the body to the neck where they empty into the veins leading to the heart. Once the debris is moved from the lymphatics to the bloodstream, it is processed and excreted from the body. These waste products include bacteria, dead white blood cells, and waste products from the cells. The lymph fluid moves through its channels by mild contractions of the lymph ducts and the surrounding skeletal muscles.

Normally the fluid moves through the channels unimpeded. However, if a person overburdens the lymph system by eating improperly or not exercising, the lymphatic fluid can accumulate and cause congestion in a particular part of the body. This was first recognized in the early 1900s by Dr. Frank Chapman, an osteopath. He discovered that when the lymphatic system is overburdened, reflex points regulating the flow of lymph turn off, shutting down the system like circuit breakers. These reflex points are located primarily on the back and chest. They are small and grainy in texture, usually no larger than a pea, and can be felt over a muscle group.

When the lymph system is overburdened, pain and congestion appear in that area. Chapman found that this correlated to organ-system and endocrine dysfunction. Firm rubbing of these points can decrease the symptoms significantly. You may want to try massaging these points, especially if the acupressure points don't work. If lymphatic congestion is the cause, pain should decrease over a few days. Locate the points on your body as indicated by the following photographs. Massage deeply and firmly with the fingers for 20 to 30 seconds.

Neurolymphatic Point 1: Beneficial Effect on Female Reproductive Organs; May Help Menopause Symptoms

Massage each area shown in the photographs for 20 to 30 seconds.

Front of the body: Area is located between the 4th and 5th ribs, behind the nipple.

Back of the body: Area is between 8th and 9th ribs, just below points of the shoulder blade.

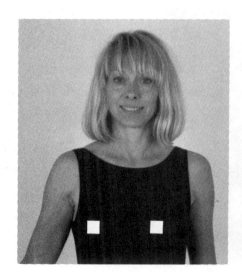
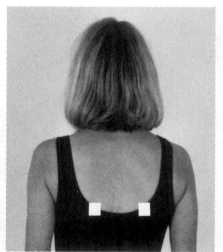

Neurolymphatic Point 2: Beneficial Effect on Female Reproductive Organs; May Help Menopausal Symptoms, Sexual Desire, and Frigidity

Massage each area shown in the photographs for 20 to 30 seconds.

Front of the body: Area is located from top of thigh bone to above knee on outside of the leg.

Back of the body: Points are on the hip bone, at the most prominent knob, at the level of L5.

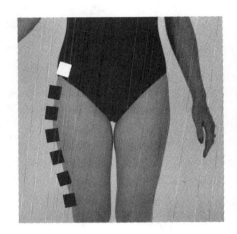
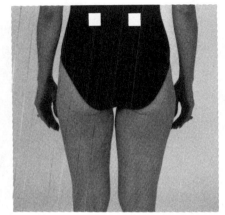

Neurolymphatic Point 3: Relieves Bladder, Lower Urinary Tract Problems

Massage each area shown in the photographs for 20 to 30 seconds.

Front of the body: Points are on either side of the navel, across the pubic bone.

Back of the body: Points are located at the lowest part of the rib cage, at L12, 1½ inches from the spine.

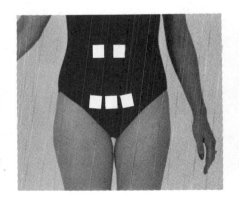
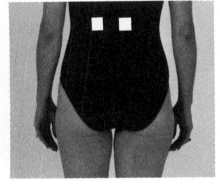

Neurolymphatic Point 4: Relieves Bladder, Lower Urinary Tract Problems

Massage each area shown in the photographs for 20 to 30 seconds.

Front of the body: Points are located along the upper and inner areas of the pubic bone.

Back of the body: Points are located at L2, one inch from the spine.

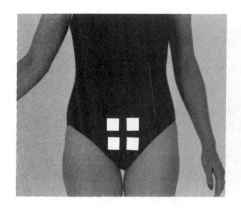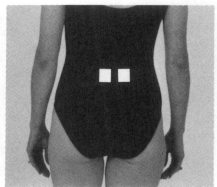

Neurolymphatic Point 5: Energizes Thyroid; Relieves Mood Swings

Massage each area shown in the photographs for 20 to 30 seconds.

Front of the body: Points are next to sternum (breast bone) between 2nd and 3rd ribs.

Back of the body: Points are located one inch from the spine between T2 and T3.

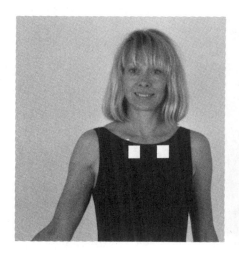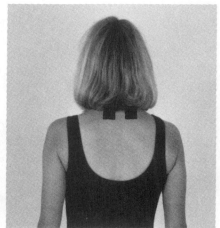

Neurolymphatic Point 6: Relieves Fatigue

Massage each area shown in the photographs for 20 to 30 seconds.

Front of the body: Points are one inch to each side of the navel and two inches above.

Back of the body: Points are located one inch from the spine between T10–11 and T11–12.

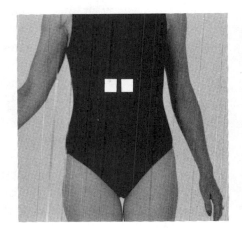
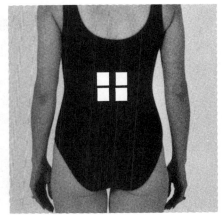

Neurolymphatic Point 7: Relieves Breast Pain and Chest Soreness

Massage each area shown on the photographs for 20 to 30 seconds.

Front of the body: Area is located along outside of legs from top of thigh to just below knee.

Back of the body: Area is located in a triangle from highest part of hip bones, L2 and L4.

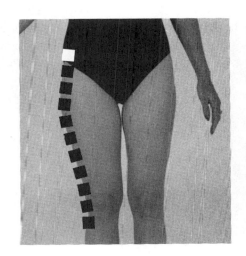
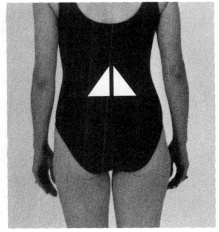

The Neurovascular Holding Points

The neurovascular holding points were discovered by Terrence Bennett, a pioneer in the field of chiropractic. He found that stimulating skin areas with light touch could improve blood circulation in deep organ systems. He observed these changes in many patients by watching their organs through a fluoroscope while pressure was being applied to their skin.

Neurovascular points are located mainly on the head. They should be touched lightly with the pads of the fingers. After holding the points for a few seconds, a slight pulsation will be felt. This pulse is not related to the heartbeat. It is thought to be the pulsation of the microcapillary bed in the skin. These points can be held from 20 seconds to 5 minutes, depending on the severity of the problem. For menopause, their greatest use is in treating symptoms related to emotional fluctuations, which can occur before and around the time of menopause.

Neurovascular Point 1: Relieves Anxiety, Mood Swings, Irritability, and Menopause Insomnia

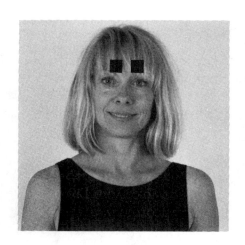

Points can be held up to 5 minutes. Concentrate on whatever feelings or situations are upsetting you. Try to feel your upset as strongly as you can. After a time, you will find that you have difficulty concentrating on the problem. It will seem to fade and you may feel much more peaceful at the end of the exercise. This is the most important exercise for relieving emotional upsets.

Frontal eminence: Located on the forehead between the eyebrows and hairline.

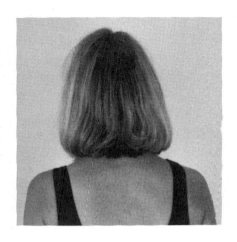

Neurovascular Point 2: Relieves Menopause Depression and Fatigue

Point can be held up to 5 minutes. Hold until negative emotion fades and energy improves.

Parietal fontanel: Located at the back of the head in the midline. This corresponds to the soft spot on the back of a baby's head.

The Right Points for Your Symptoms

The most important neurolymphatic massage points and neurovascular holding points for you are those listed next to your symptoms on the chart.

Neurolymphatic and Neurovascular Points for Menopause Symptoms

Symptoms	Neurolymphatic (NL) and Neurovascular (NV) Points
Female reproductive tract	NL-1, 2
Hot flashes	NL-1, 2
Atrophic vaginitis	NL-1, 2
Sexual desire, frigidity	NL-2
Bladder, lower urinary tract	NL-3, 4
Anxiety, irritability, insomnia	NL-5, NV-1
Depression, fatigue	NL-6, NV-2
Breast	NL-7
Thyroid	NL-5

Suggested Reading for Neurolymphatic and Neurovascular Massage:

Kapel, Priscilla. *The Body Says Yes*. ACS Publishers, 1981.

Kapel, Priscilla. *Meridian Balancing*. Self-Pub., 1979.

Peshek, Robert J. *Searching for Health, a Layman's Guide to Health Through Nutrition*. Color Coded Systems, 1982.

Thie, John F. *Touch for Health*. Pasadena, Ca.: T.H. Enterprises, 1987.

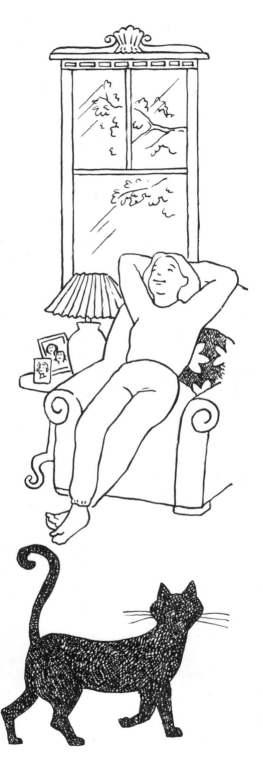

CHAPTER 16

Estrogen Replacement Therapy

Most menopausal women come up against the question of whether to use estrogen or not. There are no easy answers to this question because estrogen use has many benefits as well as risks that have to be balanced against one another when making your own decision. Even though this is a self help book, I have included this chapter on the hows and whys of estrogen therapy. As an advocate of medical self help, I believe strongly in patient education. I feel that a woman should know all the risks and benefits of any drug that she puts in her body, and have always spent a great deal of time discussing these issues with my patients. This is particularly true with estrogen replacement therapy, because you will probably use hormone therapy the rest of your life once you decide to begin taking it. This chapter should give you the information you need to make your own decision on estrogen replacement therapy as an informed patient. If you have further questions on estrogen, you should, of course, discuss them with your own physician.

Types of Estrogen

Women generally use estrogen either in pill form or as a vaginal cream. There are many brands of estrogen on the market. They are generally composed of combinations of two types of estrogens that occur naturally in your body: *estrone* and *estradiol*. Estrone is the main type of estrogen that your body makes after menopause, while Estradiol is present in greater amounts during your menstrual years. A third type of estrogen, called *estriol*, is not used in estrogen replacement pills in the United States, although research studies suggest it may be a healthier form of estrogen for women.

Both synthetic and naturally derived estrogens are available on the market. The most popular brand is Premarin (Ayerst) which is conjugated equine estrogen. It comes from the urine of pregnant mares and contains a natural mixture of estrogens including estrone. Other popular brands include Ogen (Abbott) which contains estrone, Estrace (Mead Johnson) which contains estradiol, as well as many other generic formulations. Women should avoid using the nonsteroidal estrogens. These drugs, such as diethylstilbesterol, were used several decades ago to prevent miscarriage. Unfortunately, many female children of these women have had a high incidence of vaginal and cervical abnormalities, as well as cancer. I also recommend that women avoid the estrogen pills combined with a tranquilizer such as Menrium (Roche). There are many effective, non-drug ways to combat menopause-related anxiety, such as with herbs and relaxation exercises. Tranquilizers can be habit-forming and can cause side effects like drowsiness.

How to Use Estrogen

Estrogen is usually taken as a pill. It is administered from the first to the twenty-fifth day of the month. About a week later, bleeding similar to a menstrual period will occur unless, of course, a woman has had a hysterectomy. The use of estrogen alone, however, has declined since the 1970s when medical reports indicated that women using unopposed estrogen were five times more likely to develop uterine cancer. More recent reports have shown that the addition of a progestin (progesterone-like compound) for two weeks at the end of each twenty-five-day course of estrogen appears to protect women from developing uterine cancer. As a result, most doctors today prescribe a combination of estrogen and progestin for menopause symptoms. Common brands of progestins on the market include Provera (Upjohn), Amen (Carnick), and Norlutin (Parke-Davis), among others.

Because of the possible side effects of using hormones (which I will discuss later on in this chapter), the lowest effective dose of both estrogens and progestins that relieves your symptoms should be used. Much higher doses of hormones were used several decades ago, both in estrogen replacement therapy and in birth control pills. The current trend is definitely toward using smaller doses of hormones to achieve the same beneficial effects.

Some women do not want to take the estrogen pill because it effects the entire body. If your main complaint is vaginal dryness, soreness, and painful intercourse, an estrogen cream may be used. The cream is applied to the vaginal tissues with your finger or an applicator. Estrogen creams can relieve much of the vaginal irritation that occurs with menopause due to the drop in your natural estrogen levels. Without estrogen, the vaginal lining becomes thinner, drier, and more easily traumatized. Over time, the vagina actually shrinks and becomes smaller. Within a month of using estrogen cream, many women report much greater vaginal comfort during intercourse. Although the cream is used locally, there still might be a small risk of uterine cancer and other side effects, so many doctors recommend using a course of progestins several times a year. While estrogen cream helps to decrease pain and restore the vaginal lining, the level of lubrication may not be sufficient for many women. Thus, an additional lubricant such as KY jelly may also be needed to provide extra comfort during intercourse.

Benefits of Estrogen Replacement Therapy

There are four major reasons why doctors prescribe estrogen replacement therapy for their women patients:

- Early menopause (before age 40) due to surgery
- Prevention or treatment of osteoporosis
- Elimination of hot flashes and night sweating
- Relief of vaginal dryness, soreness, and pain during intercourse.

Let's look at the beneficial effects of estrogen replacement therapy on each of these conditions.

Early menopause due to surgery. A surprising number of women under forty undergo hysterectomies for a variety of medical problems. These include pelvic infections (an increasingly common problem), cancer, endometriosis, tumors, severe bleeding, or pain due to scar tissue. Sometimes the disease process is so severe or widespread that the ovaries must be removed along with the uterus. Usually surgeons will try to leave at least one ovary or part of an ovary, since the remaining ovary will continue to secrete hormones. Sometimes this is not possible, and with the loss of both ovaries, the woman undergoes an abrupt drop in her hormone levels. Unlike the gradual drop in hormone levels that occurs with each advancing decade, this drop throws the woman's body into shock. Women report feeling hot flashes, fatigue, depression, and a loss of libido after surgery, as well as other symptoms. They are also at much greater risk of developing osteoporosis over time. For these women it is advisable to begin hormonal replacement therapy at the time of surgery. Some women elect to mimic the natural menopause reduction in hormones by decreasing hormonal doses in their forties and discontinuing hormones entirely in their fifties, while some women elect to stay on hormones indefinitely.

Prevention or treatment of osteoporosis. A number of medical studies have clearly shown that estrogen therapy decreases calcium loss from the bones after menopause. Since the effects of osteoporosis are so devastating (including loss of bone strength, thinning of bones, increased number of fractures, and poor healing of fractures), women at high risk of osteoporosis may want to consider estrogen therapy. Women at high risk include those with a family history of osteoporosis, members of an ethnic group (except African-Americans), women who are thin and short, women who have undergone menopause before forty, and women who smoke or use alcohol to excess. Estrogen replacement therapy for women at high risk of osteoporosis is even more effective when combined with calcium supplementation, vitamin D, and a regular exercise program.

Elimination of hot flashes and sweating. Estrogen is very effective in relieving hot flashes. Many women elect to use it at the time of menopause for the sake of comfort and well-being. Estrogen is not a cure, however, since the hot flashes may return once you stop using the replacement therapy. This is because your own ovaries are not revitalized or regenerated in any way by the estrogen therapy. Some medical studies have shown that vitamin E, bioflavonoids, and various herbs may also relieve hot flashes; rather than simply replacing your missing estrogen with an outside source, it is possible that these nutrients are actually stimulating your own endocrine system in some beneficial way. However, for the woman who prefers using a hormonal treatment for hot flashes, estrogen is very effective. To minimize the possibility of side effects, I generally recommend using the lowest dose that provides beneficial results.

Decrease vaginal dryness, soreness, and pain during intercourse. The drop in estrogen levels with menopause causes the vaginal walls to become thin, dry, and easily traumatized by friction. This can make intercourse uncomfortable or painful for many women. The vagina actually shrinks and becomes small without the estrogen support. Estrogen replacement therapy is very effective in building up the vaginal lining and in improving lubrication and resistance to friction. Sexual intercourse becomes much more enjoyable and comfortable with the use of estrogen replacement therapy. Some women may elect to use an estrogen cream, which may be applied directly to the vaginal tissues. This allows women to apply the exact amount that they need for relief of symptoms and may reduce the likelihood of side effects of estrogen therapy in other parts of the body.

Reasons to Avoid Estrogen

Estrogen should not be used by women at high risk of breast or uterine cancer, fibroid tumors of the uterus, endometriosis, liver or gall bladder disease, or depression. Let us look at the negative effects that estrogen can have on these medical problems.

Breast cancer. Breast cancer is one of the most common cancers of women (it is estimated that one out of eleven women will develop it during her lifetime). Many women are concerned about the connection of estrogen and cancer. While there is no strong correlation between breast cancer and estrogen replacement therapy, there may be some increased risk in women with a strong family history of breast cancer, preexisting benign breast disease, or those who develop breast lumps while on estrogen therapy. These women may decide not to use estrogen at all. If they elect to go on estrogen therapy, they should use the lowest possible dose. Women in this group should also do regular monthly breast self-examinations, and have a mammogram done every year or two as well as a breast exam by their physician.

Cancer of the uterus. Estrogen used alone was found to increase by five the number of cases of uterine cancer in the mid 1970s. Since then, it has been found that the use of progesterone with estrogen therapy seems to protect against the development of this cancer. Some women, however, may be naturally more prone to uterine cancer than others. Women who are significantly overweight (by more than 30 pounds) are at a higher risk of uterine cancer because their fat cells produce an increased amount of estrogen. These women may be advised not to use estrogen therapy, but to use instead a ten-day course of progestins to induce bleeding and shedding of the lining of the uterus.

Fibroid tumors of the uterus and endometriosis. Fibroid tumors occur when there is excessive growth in the muscular tissue of the uterus. Fibroids can grow to very large sizes in some women, enlarging the uterus to sizes seen in pregnancy. These growths are usually seen in women during their menstrual years and are stimulated by estrogen. They may expand in size with the use of estrogen-dominated birth control pills, in pregnancy, or in women who secrete high levels of estrogen naturally. Fibroids can cause excessive menstrual bleeding and pelvic discomfort to the point of necessitating a hysterectomy. Usually they shrink after menopause due to the decrease in estrogen. However, women on estrogen replacement therapy may have a continued growth of fibroid tumors. It is therefore recommended that women with active fibroid tumors avoid the use of estrogen replacement therapy. Endometriosis occurs when the lining of the uterus grows outside its normal area and implants in the pelvis. It can be responsible for pain and adhesions (scarring) in women. Growth of these implants can also be stimulated by post-menopausal hormonal therapy and this kind of therapy should be avoided.

Liver and gall bladder disease. Women with liver disease should avoid the use of estrogen replacement therapy. The liver has a key role in the chemical breakdown of estrogen and other drugs in the body so they can be safely eliminated. When the liver is compromised due to alcohol abuse, hepatitis, or other factors, it can no longer perform this function effectively.

The use of estrogen replacement therapy can also increase the risk of gall bladder disease in susceptible women. Women at risk for gall bladder disease include those who are obese, have a high-fat diet, have an elevated cholesterol level, or are diabetic. Women with a Native American ethnic background also run a high risk of gall bladder disease and should not use estrogen replacement therapy.

Depression and mood changes. Some women find that hormonal replacement therapy improves their mood tremendously, while others find that estrogen replacement therapy and progestins can cause depression and mood changes. Interestingly enough, mood changes can also be seen with the birth control pill. In fact, younger women are usually warned that mood changes can occur. If this happens, they are either changed to another birth control pill or are taken off oral contraceptives altogether.

Heart disease and high blood pressure. The evidence that hormonal therapy increases the risk of heart disease, strokes, and elevated blood pressure is contradictory at the present time. Some studies show an increased risk of circulatory disease while using hormonal therapy, while other studies report a reduction in the risk of heart disease and hypertension. As a general rule, women who have a higher risk of cardiovascular disease should be monitored more closely while on estrogen replacement therapy, or should not use hormonal therapy at all. This includes women who have diabetes, elevated blood pressure, high cholesterol levels, smoke to excess, or are prone to obesity. If you have any of these risk factors and are considering estrogen replacement therapy, it is important to discuss your own situation with your doctor to see if replacement therapy would be indicated or not.

Because the risk of cardiovascular disease increases in the older population, special note should be taken of any possible symptoms of circulatory disease that can occur while using estrogen replacement therapy. These symptoms include blurred vision, chest pain, numbness or weakness in any part of your body, or any abrupt rise in blood pressure. If you notice any of these symptoms, notify your doctor immediately.

Common Estrogens Used for Hormonal Replacement Therapy

Brand Name	Generic Name
DES	diethylstilbestrol
Estinyl	ethinyl estradiol
Estrace	estradiol
Ogen	estrone
Premarin	conjugated equine estrogens
Menrium	esterified estrogens and librium
Tace	chlorotrianisene

Common Progestins Used for Hormonal Replacement Therapy

Brand Name	Generic Name
Provera	Medroxyprogesterone acetate
Amen	Medroxyprogesterone acetate
Norlutin	Norethindrone
Norlutate	Norethindrone acetate

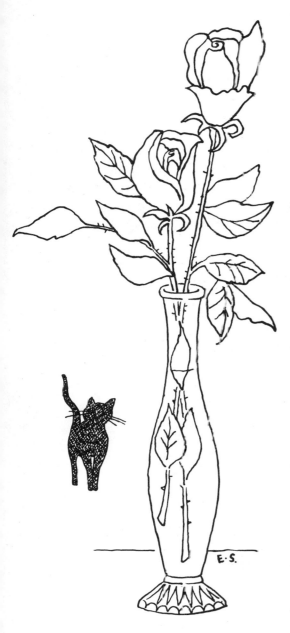

CHAPTER 17

Putting Your Program Together

The *Menopause Self Help Book* gives you a complete program to help relieve some of your menopause symptoms and to prevent others, and to attain new levels of health and vitality. The self help program contains a great many treatment options. Try them and see which techniques work best for you. The Complete Treatment Chart on pages 32–35 should help you put together your own program simply and easily. It emphasizes all the main points that I would like you to keep in mind. Don't get bogged down in details. Always keep in mind your ultimate objective: relief of menopause symptoms and improvement in your overall health. The goal is to get stronger and healthier as you age. As you learn new techniques of wellness, your health can actually improve as you get older.

Enjoy the program and use it as a new and exciting learning experience. Have fun with the exercises. Treat the changes in your dietary habits as an opportunity to try delicious new foods.

Healing occurs in a stepwise progression. It is never a straight line. Don't feel guilty if you miss a day of exercises. Don't become discouraged if you go off your diet for holidays, vacations, or just because your old food cravings become too strong. Everyone falls down at times. The successful person picks herself up and moves on. Just keep going back to your goals periodically and review the general guidelines that I've outlined for you.

Be your own best feedback system. Become sensitive to your

body's messages. Your body will tell you when certain foods or emotional stress may worsen your symptoms.

Remember that even moderate changes in your habits can improve your health and help to prevent many of the symptoms that we call "the aging process." Problems such as stiffness, lack of flexibility, and fatigue, as well as many illnesses, can be prevented or decreased in severity with proper attention to preventive health care techniques. A strong and healthy body can and should be a lifelong goal.

Nutrition

Make all nutritional changes gradually. Review periodically the lists of foods to limit and foods to emphasize. Each time you review this list, pick several more foods that you are willing to eliminate and some to try. Review these lists as often as you choose, but try to do it on a regular basis. Every small change that you make in your diet can help.

Review the guidelines for each meal. You may want to restructure a particular meal. The sample menus that I've provided in the text can serve as models for you.

Use vitamin and herbal supplements to help round out your nutritional needs. Menopause is a time when your body needs more nutrients to remain optimally healthy.

Stress Reduction

The exercises in the stress reduction chapter can be very helpful if you are sensitive to both the hormonal and emotional changes that occur with menopause. The menopause stress-reduction exercises can help to balance your mood and enhance your sense of well-being. They will also help to change your belief system about your body as well as improve your autonomic nervous system function.

When you begin your program, set aside half an hour for several consecutive days and try all the stress-reduction exercises described in this book. Find the combination that works for you and then practice it regularly.

The exercises should be done on a daily basis for at least a few minutes a day. You may find that the best times to practice them are when you wake up in the morning or at night before you go to sleep. Other useful times are during the day when you are feeling particularly frazzled or stressed. Simply take ten minutes, close the door to your room, and relax. Breathe deeply, meditate, or use the menopause visualizations or affirmations. You will find that you feel much better afterward. You may also find that you enjoy doing the stress-reduction exercises before doing your regular physical exercise.

Exercise

Moderate exercise—walking, jogging, swimming, golf, playing tennis, or bicycling—should be done on a regular basis along with the fitness and flexibility exercises. Every day or every other day is best, depending on your tolerance level.

Specific Corrective Exercises: Acupressure Massage, Yoga, Neurolymphatic Points, Neurovascular Holding Points

The first week or two, set aside half an hour to an hour a day for several consecutive days and do the exercises that warm up, tone, and energize the body. Find the ones you enjoy the most. These should always precede any specific corrective exercises for your symptoms.

Look up the specific exercises that will correct your symptoms on the Complete Treatment Chart on pages 32–35. Try out all the exercises for your specific symptoms. Find the ones that work best for you. Practice them on a regular basis so that they help to prevent and relieve your symptoms.

Workbook Section

Fill out the workbook section before you begin your program. Then, use it periodically (every 1 to 3 months) to see the progress you are making as well as the problem areas where you need to spend more time. Regular use of the workbook section will make the program much easier and more effective for you.

The workbook pages give you a structured format with which to evaluate your habit patterns, your symptoms, and your success. The habit evaluation section will show you which areas of your life contribute to your symptoms. Check off your menopause symptoms and list which treatments you are doing to help correct them. It is important that you give yourself this feedback in an organized and easy-to-use format.

Conclusion

As I finish this book, I want to leave you with several thoughts. Remember that menopause and the years beyond can be a time of vigor and vitality. Getting older can give you the opportunity to learn new techniques of health maintenance. Many women pay more attention to their lifestyle habits in the menopause years and, consequently, enjoy better health than they did when they were younger. This learning process can be an exciting adventure which will add to your joy of living. It certainly has added to mine!

So, practice the menopause self help techniques in this book on a daily basis. Practice good nutritional habits, relaxation and stress techniques, adequate exercise, and any specific corrective techniques that help to relieve your specific symptoms. If you master them and make them part of your everyday life, you will be rewarded with the same wonderful results that my patients and I have had. They will provide the basis for a healthy, enjoyable life.

APPENDIX:

Additional Self Help Resources

Health Publications

Healthletters
Santa Fe Health Education Project
P.O. Box 577
Santa Fe, NM 87504
(505) 982-3236
    Bilingual (English/Spanish) health information
for women.

HotFlash: A Newsletter for Midlife and Older Women
c/o National Action Forum for Midlife
    and Older Women
Box 816
Stony Brook, NY 11790-0609
    Contains articles and news about health and social
issues. Quarterly. $15 per year.

Medical Self Care
P.O. Box 717
Inverness, CA 94937
    A quarterly magazine on all aspects of health,
self-care, consumer-oriented medicine.

Midlife Wellness Center for Climacteric Studies
University of Florida
901 NW 8th Ave., Suite B1
Gainesville, FL 32601
    A quarterly journal on all aspects of the menopause
and aging for health professionals and the general
public.

National Women's Health Network
1325 G St., NW
Lower Level
Washington, DC 20005
(202) 347-1140
    Monthly newsletter and various health
publications, $25 membership.

Nutrition Action Center for Science in the Public
Interest
1501 Sixteenth St., NW
Washington, DC 20036
  A monthly magazine on practical nutritional
  information and the political battles for
  consumer education about food and health.

Radiance
P.O. Box 31703
Oakland, CA 94604
(415) 482-0680
  Quarterly national magazine for women of all
  sizes, ages, and lifestyles. Offers resources and
  information for all areas of life. $12 per year.

Roundtable Report
1718 Connecticut Ave., NW #310
Washington, DC 20009
(202) 328-1415
  Publication (11 issues/year) on women's health care
  published by Federation of Organizations for
  Professional Women. $25 per year.

Wise Women Center
P.O. Box 64, Dept. HRD
Woodstock, NY 12498
(914) 246–8081
  Workshops and apprenticeships in herbal medicine
  and healing in the Wise Woman tradition. Free
  brochure.

Womenwise
38 S. Main St.
Concord, NH 03301
(603) 225-2739
  Quarterly tabloid published by the New
  Hampshire Feminist Center. $7.

Health Organizations

Alcoholics Anonymous
General Service Office
Box 459, Grand Central Station
New York, NY 10163
(212) 686-1100

American Cancer Society (National Headquarters)
1599 Clifton Rd., NE
Atlanta, GA 30329
(800) ACS-2345

American Diabetes Association
National Service Center
1660 Duke St.
Alexandria, VA 22314
(800) 232-3472

Arthritis Foundation
1314 Spring St., NW
Atlanta, GA 30309
(404) 872-7100

Berkeley Women's Health Clinic
2908 Ellsworth St.
Berkeley, CA 94705
(415) 843-6194

Boston Women's Healthbook Collective
47 Nichols Ave.
Watertown, MA 02172
(617) 924-0271
  Dedicated to women's health information
  and services, including the Women's Health
  Information Center.

Breast Cancer Advisory Center
11426 Rockville Pike, Suite 406
Rockville, MD 20850
(301) 984-1040

Committee for Freedom of Choice in Cancer Therapy
1180 Walnut Ave.
Chula Vista, CA 92011
(619) 429-8200

Foundation for Advancement in Cancer Therapy
P.O. Box 1242 Old Chelsea Station
New York, NY 10011
(212) 741-2790

National Council on Alcoholism, Inc.
12 West 21st St., 8th Floor
New York, NY 10010
(212) 206-6770

National Hospice Organization
1901 N Ft. Myer
Arlington, VA 22209
  Hospice resources.

Women's Occupational Health Resource Center
School of Public Health
600 West 168th St.
New York, NY 10032

Y-Me
1757 Ridge Road
Homewood, IL 60430
  Education, counseling, and referrals for women
  with breast cancer.

Activist Publications and Sources

Common Woman Books
8724 109th St.
Edmonton, Alberta T6G 1E9
Canada
(403) 432-9344
  Feminist bookstore. Will mail lists of books
  available in your area of interest.

Feminist Collections
729 State St. #112A Memorial Library
(608) 263-5754
Madison, WI 53706
  Various feminist publications published by
  University of Wisconsin. Bibliographies available
  on topics of interest.

Feminist Studies
University of Maryland
College Park, MD 20742
(301) 454-2363
  Tri-annual publication published by University of
  Maryland. Commentaries, analysis, and directions
  for research and action. $18 per year.

Heresies
P.O. Box 1306, Canal Street Station
New York, NY 10017
(212) 227-2108
  A biannual feminist publication on art and politics.
  Longest running feminist art magazine in U.S.
  Four-issue subscription $23.

National Now Times
1000 16th St., NW
Washington, DC 20036
(202) 331-0066
  Women's tabloid (6 issues/year) published by the
  National Organization for Women (NOW). $35 per
  year.

National Women's Mailing List
P.O. Box 68
Jenner, CA 95450
(707) 632-5763
  Maintains a 60,000-name network of feminists
  interested in a wide variety of women's issues.

Off Our Backs
1841 Columbia Rd., NW, #217
Washington, DC 20009
(202) 234-8072
Respected feminist newspaper (11 issues/year). Wide range of topics: articles, arts, reviews, and reports on conferences. $11 per year.

Plainswoman
P.O. Box 8027
Grand Forks, ND 58202
(701) 777-8043
Feminist publication (10 issues/year) for Midwest women. $15 per year.

Sojourner: The Women's Forum
143 Albany St.
Cambridge, MA 02139
Feminist monthly newspaper. $15 per year.

The Brown Papers
P.O. Box 50583
Washington, DC 20004
Quarterly report on contributions made by women of many minorities. $15 per year.

Woman of Power
P.O. Box 827
Cambridge, MA 02238
Quarterly national magazine integrating spiritual, cultural, and feminist issues. $18 per year.

WomaNews
P.O. Box 220 Village Station
New York, NY 10014
(212) 989-7963
Comprehensive women's tabloid (10 issues/year), $8.

Activist Organizations

Grandmothers for Peace
909 12th St., Suite 118
Sacramento, CA 95814
(916) 444-5080
Dedicated to halting nuclear arms race; open to all.

League of Women Voters
1730 M St., NW
Washington, DC 20036
(202) 429-1965
Encourages informed participation of citizens in government. Membership is open to all.

Legal Services Corporation
400 Virginia Ave., SW
Washington, DC 20024-2751
(202) 863-1820

National Council of Senior Citizens
925 15th St., NW
Washington, DC 20005
(202) 347-8800

National Organization for Women (NOW)
1401 New York Ave., NW, Suite 800
Washington, DC 20005

National Self-Help Clearinghouse
33 West 42nd St.
New York, NY 10036
(212) 642-2944

National Senior Citizens' Law Center
2025 M St., NW, Suite 400
Washington, DC 20036
(202) 887-5280
Operates a legal services support center and advocates for poor elderly clients.

National Women's Political Caucus (NWPC)
1275 K St., NW, Suite 750
Washington, DC 20005
(202) 898-1100
   NWPC's goal is to get more women elected and
   appointed to political office.

Peace Links
747 8th St., SE
Washington, DC 20003
(202) 544-0805
   Grassroots organization of mainstream women
   dedicated to mobilizing people against nuclear war.
   Excellent information kits available.

The Villers Foundation
1334 G St., NW
Washington, DC 20005
(202) 628-3030
   Provides financial support and assistance for
   projects aimed at empowerment of older persons.
   Write for their list of publications.

Spiritual Publications and Organizations

Celibate Women
3306 Ross Pl., NW
Washington, DC 20008
(202) 966-7783
   Biannual journal about the positive aspects of
   voluntary celibacy for women.

Feminist Spiritual Community
P.O. Box 3771
Portland, ME 04104

GAIA Bookstore & Catalog Company
1400 Shattuck Ave., Store #10
Berkeley, CA 94709
(415) 548-4172
   Bookstore, resource center, and catalog company
   celebrating women, the earth, and feminine
   spirituality. To receive last catalog, send $1.

National Council of Jewish Women
53 West 23rd St.
New York, NY 10010
(212) 532-1740

National Interfaith Coalition on Aging
P.O. Box 1924
298 South Hull St.
Athens, GA 30603
(404) 353-1331

Reclaiming: Center for Feminist Spirituality
P.O. Box 14404
San Francisco, CA 94144

Spiritual Women's Times
P.O. Box 51186
Seattle, WA 98115-1186
   Quarterly women's spirituality newspaper. Annual
   subscription $7.50.

Mature Woman

American Association of Retired Persons (AARP)
1909 K St., NW
Washington, DC 20049
(202) 872-4700

Gray Panthers
311 South Juniper St., Suite 601
Philadelphia, PA 19107
(215) 545-6555

National Council on the Aging (NCOA)
600 Maryland Ave., SW, West Wing 100
Washington, DC 20024
(202) 479-1200

Options for Women Over Forty
3543 18th St.
San Francisco, CA 94110
(415) 431-6405
 Support and counseling for mid-life women.

Vintage 45
165 Overhill Rd.
Orinda, CA 94563
(415) 254-7266
 Quarterly mature woman's journal. $8.40 per year.

Work-Professional

Feminist Teacher
Ballantine 442, Indiana University
Bloomington, IN 47405
 Quarterly magazine for teachers, from
 preschool to the universities. $12 per year.

Minerva
1101 S. Arlington Ridge Rd., #210
Arlington, VA 22202
(703) 892-4388
 Quarterly magazine for military, defense, and
 governmentally employed women. $20 per year.

National Business Woman
2012 Massachusetts Ave., NW
Washington, DC 20036
(202) 293-1100
 Quarterly magazine about career developments.
 $10 per year.

9 to 5 Newsletter
614 Superior Ave., NW
Cleveland, OH 44113
(216) 566-9308
 Bimonthly respected women's newsletter covering
 legislation, working conditions, resources for
 networking, and issues concerning older women
 and minorities. $25 per year.

NOW Legal Defense and Education Fund
99 Hudson St.
New York, NY 10013
(212) 925-6635

Older Women's League (OWL)
730 11th St., NW, Suite 300
Washington, DC 20001
(202) 783-6686

Savvy Magazine
P.O. Box 6048
Palm Coast, FL 32037
 Monthly magazine for businesswomen.

Successful Woman
1511 Walnut St.
Philadelphia, PA 19102
(215) 563-4415
 Monthly newsletter for women focusing on laws,
 taxes, finances, career development, education,
 and more. $42 per year.

The Executive Female
127 West 24th St.
Fourth Floor
New York, NY 10011
(212) 645-0770
 Bimonthly magazine published by the National
 Association for Female Executives. Reviews,
 profiles, financial planning, career development,
 and calendar. Membership $29 per year.

Women's Equity Action League (WEAL)
1250 I St., NW, Suite 305
Washington, DC 20005
(202) 898-1588
   WEAL promotes economic equity for women
   through legislation, litigation, and public
   education.

Women's Yellow Pages
P.O. Box 66093
Los Angeles, CA 90066
(213) 398-5761

Working Woman
P.O. Box 10132
Des Moines, IA 50340
(515) 247-7500
   Monthly magazine covering a wide range of topics.
   $18 per year.

Recreational

Eve's Garden
119 West 57th St., #1406
New York, NY 10019
(212) 757-8651
   Women's erotic mail-order catalog. $1.

Fighting Woman News
P.O. Box 1459 Grand Central Station
New York, NY 10163
   Quarterly publication on sports and martial arts
   for women.

Kalliope
3939 Roosevelt Blvd.
Jacksonville, FL 32205
(904) 387-8211
   A journal of women's art.

Ladyslipper
P.O. Box 3130
Durham, NC 27705
(919) 683-1570
   Free mail-order catalog includes music supplies,
   calendars, cards and posters, etc.

Womantrek-Worldwide Travel
P.O. Box 20643
Seattle, WA 98102
(206) 325-4772
   International adventures for women of all ages and
   physical ability. Safaris, rafting, trekking, bicycle
   tours, etc.

The PMS and Menopause Self Help Center

The PMS and Menopause Self Help Center
101 First Street, Suite 441
Los Altos, CA 94022
For Appointments and Information: (415) 964-7268
For Orders: (415) 964-7268
Susan M. Lark, M.D., Director
Christine Green, M.D., Director of Patient Education

The PMS and Menopause Self Help Center has many helpful resources and activities for women. We provide a professional registry and nationwide referral and information network for women needing support groups, physicians, nurse practitioners, and clinics in their area. We also give PMS and menopause workshops and seminars in different parts of the country. Please let us know if this is of interest to you or your group.

Our resources for women include our two books—*The PMS Self Help Book* and *The Menopause Self Help Book*—as well as our booklets on anemia and heavy menstrual flow, menstrual cramps, chronic fatigue, and breast cysts and cancer (all of which contain self help programs and helpful information by Dr. Lark), *and* nutritional systems (vitamins, minerals, and herbs) for PMS, menopause, sleep/ relaxation, 30-day cycle normalizer, menstrual cramps, general women's formula, and hematinic (for anemia). We also have stress reduction audio tapes.

Dr. Lark sees women patients in her private practice in Los Altos. She is also available for phone consultation sessions. While she cannot diagnose or treat conditions by phone, many women have questions about such topics as vitamins, herbs, food choices, and setting up their own home program. Please call Dr. Lark at (415) 964-7268 for more information or to set up an appointment.

Index

About Susan M. Lark, M.D.

Susan M. Lark, M.D., is a noted authority in women's health care and preventive medicine. She is the Director of The PMS and Menopause Self Help Center in Los Altos. She also see patients in her private practice in Los Altos. Dr. Lark has been on the clinical faculty of Stanford University Medical School, Department of Family and Preventive Medicine. She is an associate member of the Department of Family Medicine, El Camino Hospital in Mountain View, California. Dr. Lark lectures widely on women's health issues, and is the author of *The PMS Self Help Book* (Celestial Arts), the best-selling guide for women with PMS. Dr. Lark can be reached through The PMS and Menopause Self Help Center, for women wishing to see her for patient care or for lectures and speaking engagements. She is also available for phone consultation for women who would like more personalized information and do not live in the San Francisco Bay Area. Dr. Lark can be contacted for available times and fee schedule through the Center at (415) 964-7268.

Information for ordering additional products developed by Susan M. Lark, M.D.

Dr. Susan Lark's books and nutritional systems for women are available from The PMS and Menopause Self Help Center, 101 First Street, Suite 441, Los Altos, CA 94022-2706. Call (415) 964-7268 (for information), or (800) 862-9876 (for orders only). Major credit cards accepted.

Books by Susan M. Lark, M.D.
PMS Self Help Book
Menopause Self Help Book
Anemia and Heavy Bleeding—A Self Help Program
Menstrual Cramps—A Self Help Program
Chronic Fatigue and Tiredness—A Self Help Program

Tapes
PMS Stress Reduction Tape

Foods
Flax Oil
Flax Oil Capsules
Flax Seed Powder
Vegelicious Non-Dairy Milk

Vitamin and Mineral Supplements Formulated Specifically for Women
PMS Nutritional System
Menopause Nutritional System
Women's Daily Spectrum Nutritional System
Women's Daily Iron Nutritional System
Women's Energy and Vitality Nutritional System
Bioflavonoids

Herbal Tinctures for Women

Yellow Dock	Ginger Root
Huckleberry	White Willow Bark
Oregon Grape Root	Red Raspberry Leaf
Tumeric	Cramp Bark
Wild Yam	Chamomile
Shepherd's Purse	Hops
Goldenseal	Chaste Tree Berry
Sarsaparilla	Gingko Biloba
Black Cohosh	Parsley
Buchu	

Recipe Cards and Meal Plans

Recipe Cards and Meal Plans for Healthy Women—Breakfast

Recipe Cards and Meal Plans for Healthy Women—Lunch and Dinner

Recipe Cards and Meal Plans for Healthy Women—Snacks and Desserts

Women's Personal Products

Vitamin E Vaginal Suppositories

Products for Muscle Tension and Back Discomfort

The Archable Body Bridge

ORDER FORM

Charge It! If you have a VISA or MasterCard, you can charge your order. Call toll-free 1-800-862-9876. LifeCycles' phone order center is open from 8am to 9pm, Eastern Time, Monday through Friday.

Because we anticipate that you will be using this book for many years to come, it is likely that prices will change and new items will be added from time to time. Therefore, we have not included prices for the items that LifeCycles stocks. Please call our toll-free number, 1-800-862-9876 for current prices, new products, and any specials that LifeCycles may have at the time of your order.

If you wish to order by mail, please follow the 4 steps in numerical order to complete this form. Make sure to follow all the steps, and then to sign the form in the space provided. Mail completed forms to: LifeCycles, 101 First Street, Suite 441, Los Altos, CA 94022-2706.

1. ORDERED BY

Name

Address

City   State/Province   Zip/Postal Code

Daytime Phone Number (Area Code First)

Order Date (Month/Day/Year)

2. METHOD OF PAYMENT

☐ MasterCard   ☐ VISA   ☐ Check or Money Order

Card Number

Expiration Date (Month/Year)

Your Signature   Dated

3. SHIP TO (if different from "Ordered By" address)

Name

Address

City   State/Province   Zip/Postal Code

4. ITEMS AVAILABLE TO ORDER

(Please note that these are the items available to order from LifeCycles at the time of this book's printing. Books, products available and prices are subject to change. Use this form to note the items and quantities you wish to order, and then call LifeCycles toll-free at 1-800-862-9876 to get prices and complete your order.)

A. BOOKS BY SUSAN M. LARK, M.D.

NO.	DESCRIPTION	QTY.	PRICE
1A.	PMS Self-Help Book		
2A.	Menopause Self Help Book		
3A.	Anemia & Heavy Menstrual Flow: A Self-Help Program		
4A.	Menstrual Cramps: A Self-Help Program		
5A.	Chronic Fatigue & Tiredness: A Self-Help Program		

B. NUTRITIONAL PRODUCTS

NO.	DESCRIPTION	QTY.	PRICE
1B.	PMS Vitamin Supplement		
2B.	PMS Herbal Supplement		
3B.	PMS Nutritional System (Combines 1B & 2B)		
4B.	Menopause Vitamin Supplement		
5B.	Menopause Herbal Supplement		
6B.	Menopause Nutritional System (Combines 4B & 5B)		
7B.	Daily Iron Product		
8B.	Daily Spectrum Supplement		

C. OTHER PRODUCTS

LifeCycles also features food products, skin care products, audio and video tapes, personal products and other items. Write or call LifeCycles toll-free 1-800-862-9876 for a free brochure, or ask your LifeCycles phone rep for details when you call.

More useful books...

THE PMS SELF-HELF BOOK by Susan Lark, M.D.
A wonderful hands-on workbook that helps women identify the causes of common PMS symptoms (anxiety, pain, weight gain, chocolate craving, etc.) and diminish or eliminate them through diet, exercise, acupressure, and other drug-free methods. $16.95. paper, 240 pages.

WOMEN'S INTUITION by Elizabeth Davis.
"*Women's Intuition* is a delight. Davis shows how biological events in women's lives influence intuitive capacities. A gentle and strengthening companion...(this book) left me feeling confirmed in my own journey as a woman."--*East West* magazine
An examination of intuition in women's lives, and how it can be used to help solve problems, make decisions, and deal with personal relationships. $7.95 paper, 112 pages.

GENTLE YOGA by Lorna Bell, R.N. and Eudora Seyfer.
This book is especially designed for people with arthritis, stroke damage, or multiple sclerosis, those in wheelchairs, or anyone who needs a gentle, practical way to improve their health through exercise. The book is spiralbound to stay open while you work and includes over 135 helpful illustrations. $12.95 spiral, 144 pages, $8.95 paper.

HEADACHES: The Drugless Way to Lasting Relief by Harry Ehrmantraut, Ph.D.
How to overcome tension headaches, migraines, and headaches caused by allergies, caffeine, hangover, and depression—without drugs. $8.95 paper, 152 pages.

GREATER ENERGY AT YOUR FINGERTIPS by Michael Reed Gach.
Based on Chinese breathing exercise and acupressure points, these easy-to-do exercises effectively increase your energy—in just ten minutes a day. Over 150 photos demonstrate how to reduce stress and fatigue and boost vitality. $8.95 paper, 160 pages.

THE SERPENT AND THE WAVE by Jalaja Bonheim.
Many cultures consider dance and movement to be sacred arts, but Westerners have long ignored the power and wisdom of their bodies. This book, by a professional dancer and teacher of movement meditation, gives a fresh, new, Western approach to improving body image and gaining control through simple, well-illustrated exercises and affirmations. $14.95 paper, 320 pages.

WELLNESS...Small Changes That You Can Use To Make A Big Difference by John Travis, M.D. and Regina Ryan. Geared to busy people, or those who are not ready to radically change their lifestyle, this book outlines fifty small changes anyone can make in areas including nutrition, relaxation, work, and relationships. The suggestions can be taken together to form a coherent wellness program, or done one at a time as convenient.
$5.95 paper, 80 pages. A TEN SPEED PRESS BOOK

WELLNESS WORKBOOK by John Travis, M.D. and Regina Ryan.
An updated editon of one of the first books on total wellness—how to integrate physical, emotional, intellectual, and spiritual factors to create vibrant, life-long health. $13.95 paper, 256 pages. A TEN SPEED PRESS BOOK

Available from your local bookstore, or order direct from the publisher. Please include $2.50 shipping & handling for the first book, and 50 cents for each additional book. California residents include local sales tax. Write for our free complete catalog of over 400 books and tapes.

Ship to:
Name_____
Address_____
City _____ State _____ Zip _____
Phone:(___)_____

CELESTIAL ARTS
Box 7123
Berkeley, CA 94707
For VISA or MasterCard orders call (800) 841-BOOK